YOGA

An Analytical Release

Physical fitness and relief alone are poor bargains!

Yoga can banish misery rooted in our way of thinking.

It exposes life as quasi, virtual

and blurs friend-foe, own-alien distinctions!

by Hardev S. Thakur

Note for Librarians: A cataloguing record for this book is available from Library and Archives Canada at www.collectionscanada.ca/amicus/index-e.html
ISBN 1-4251-0833-4

TRAFFORD PUBLISHING

Offices in Canada, USA, Ireland and UK

Book sales for North America and international:
Trafford Publishing, 6E–2333 Government St.,
Victoria, BC V8T 4P4 CANADA
phone 250 383 6864 (toll-free 1 888 232 4444)
fax 250 383 6804; email to orders@trafford.com
Book sales in Europe:
Trafford Publishing (UK) Limited, 9 Park End Street, 2nd Floor
Oxford, UK OX1 1HH UNITED KINGDOM
phone +44 (0)1865 722 113 (local rate 0845 230 9601)
facsimile +44 (0)1865 722 868; info.uk@trafford.com
Order online at:
trafford.com/06-2591

10 9 8 7 6 5 4 3 2

YOGA
AN ANALYTICAL RELEASE

by Hardev S. Thakur

Dedicated to:

My Parents and Teachers
&
People appreciative of Him in all and
serving all even if at own expense

CONTENTS

ABBREVIATIONS AND NOTATIONS

Refer to Transliteration Key[1] and Glossary (Appendix A).

AU	...	The Aitareya (āiṭa-) Upanishad
BG	...	The Bhagavad (-ḍ) Gita (gīṭā), or The Gita
BS	...	The Brahma Sutras or Vedanta Sutras
BU	...	The Brihadaranyaka (bṛhaḍāraṇyaka) Upanishad
CU	...	The Chhandogya (-ānḍog-) Upanishad
IU	...	The Isha (īśā) Upanishad (or the XL hymn of YV)
KU	...	The Katha Upanishad
KVU	...	The Kaivalya Upanishad
MB	...	The Mahabharata (mahābhāraṭa), an epic
MU	...	The Mandukya (māṇḍūkya) Upanishad
RV	...	The Rig (ṛg) Veda
US	...	Upadesasahasri (upaḍeśasāhasrī), Book of Thousand Advices, by Advaita Vedanta (non-dualist) philosopher Shankara
YS/Yoga		Yoga Sutras of Patanjali
YV	...	The Yajur Veda (White)

In case of Yoga (yoga sutras), references will simply be made like **I 2** — Roman numeral will indicate chapter (Quarter) number, and Hindu-Arabic numeral the sutra number. References for other books would be like **BG III 5**.

---

1 **a** (org*a*n), **ā** (f*a*ther), **i** (p*i*n), **ī** (p*i*que), **u** (p*u*ll), **ū** (r*u*le), **ṛ** (fib*re*), **e** (th*ey*), and **o** (b*o*ne)
b, **h**, **j**, **k**, **l**, **m**, **n**, **p**, **r**, **s**, **v**, and **y** have usual English values; **g** as in *g*old;
j (*j*ug), **ch** (*ch*ur*ch*), and **ś** (*sh*ip) involve similar oral effort (*palatal*);
t, **d**, **ṣ** (sh), **ṇ** are uttered with retroflexed tongue (*lingual*);
ṭ, **ṭh** (*th*in), **ḍ** (*th*en), and **ḍh** (wi*thh*old) are *dental* sounds;
ḥ indicates aspiration; **ň**, **ñ**, **ṇ**, **n**, **m**, and **ṃ** indicate nasal sounds;
bh (jo*b h*ouse), **dh** (a*dh*ere), and so on. *Hints are provided in parentheses and footnotes.*

No one is really working for peace unless he is
working primarily for the restoration of wisdom.

[*E. F. Schumacher*]

PREFACE

Yogi

AT PEACE WITH HIMSELF AND WORLD

Word yoga evokes in us a host of emotions *viz.* wonder, fascination, awe, mystery, and even greed. …

And word yogi[2] brings to our mind stories about some ones unknown, living in far-off places, avoiding the hustle of life for meditation; following austere routines; and capable of performing miracles. …

Thus, yoga can look evasive, contradictory, and perplexing! And yogi, from others' standpoint, can look to be leading a paradoxical life! For instance, on one hand, he possesses miracle-producing powers and, on the other, practises self-rejection and self-denial. Possessing powers of no use to oneself is meaningless.

The above account is incoherent and lacking. … Yoga is esoteric! … There are no inconsistencies and pretensions in life of yoga. Whereas life that others lead is contradictory and paradoxical, *e.g.*, people do not live up to their preaching and projected image.

Yogi truly leads a simple and unassuming life. He neither lives in charted conditions nor rejects and escapes life. Rather the way HE ENJOYS THE AVAILABLE (IN FULL AWARENESS) others do not and even cannot visualise the qualitative

---

[2] Yogi is a Sanskrit word used for someone male who has unflinching commitment to yoga. For female, the word used is yogini. Word yogin can be used for either.

difference. Yogi is at peace with himself and with world at large. ...

The secret of his joy is that he does not seek pleasure and powers and not even virtue and knowledge. His mind is so resolved that HE DOES NOT SEEK ENJOYMENT OUTSIDE [OR IN NON-SELF].[3] Free from capricious impulses and mental traps[4], he enjoys true liberation. ... To others such life can look austere and monotonous. Whereas, from the perspective of yogi, others spend themselves in wild goose chase [greed] of objects of desire.[5] It is a wild goose chase because there is no way to grasp things – that is what *Viveka* (Discrimination) signifies. Grasping is a perception, an illusion! Alternatively, *upalabdhi* [a façade of gain]!

Therefore, if reader is drawn to yoga out of greed, their greed should vanish by the time they finish the book. That should happen because they are by that time expected to have realised the agony of greed – no matter what the object of greed is! GREED ITSELF IS EVIL – ignorance-in-action (Tamas-Rajas combo). WATCH AGAINST **TRISHNA** (तृष्णा – greed, or desire for more), which is insatiable and keeps surfacing in infinite forms. It remains the prime target of Yoga (the source book on yoga[6]). This can be noticed in Yoga [I 15-16] when the two types of detachment are explained. Love of power and status is no-no; Yoga expressly cautions against greedy satisfaction and interest in allurements and temptations. Otherwise, evil can re-emerge. [III 51]

It is not amazing if this book skips discussion on powers, which form the third chapter of Yoga called Glory (Vibhuti).

---

[3] Of course, inside too there is no need to seek. Pleasure and powers are natural offshoots of yoga.

[4] Refer to opening sutra of Synopsis.

[5] Objects are not consumed; we indeed get spent and die. Face has got badly wrinkled; hair gone grey; organs worn out and loose – Trishna alone remains youthful. (Bhartrihari)

[6] By yoga (with y small) we mean the discipline and philosophy; and by Yoga, *Yoga Sutras of Patanjali* that comprises sutras (aphorisms) on yoga written by Sage Patanjali.

Yoga

Yoga (योग) is a dynamic philosophy.

It is not just physical workout – latter being only peripheral. If Yoga prescribes Asana and Pranayama, that is to ensure a supportive physico-psychologically fit vehicle [body] for yoga. However, why call it supportive and not essential? Metaphysical explanation is that activity (*rajas*) is used to overcome inertia (*tamas*) – inertia is fundamental to matter of which our body is made. Next, why call peripheral? The explanation is that Yoga itself calls it so. [III 7-8] In addition, illness, laziness, et al (mentioned in the Synopsis) distract only apparently and temporarily; they do not debar one from yoga.

It is commonly believed that yoga means union or unification. But it is not so. If it were, then it must have a beginning at some point of time and then, unfortunately, fear and possibility of break-up at some point later. Where there is beginning, there is end too! In that case, yoga eventually cannot provide a durable remedy! ... Yoga must therefore be an INTRINSIC UNION and not an arranged one.

Yoga is an EFFORTLESS way of life [*being*] and not a life of our making or choice [*becoming*]. ... Understandably, then, actions whether moral or immoral cannot defile anyone! ...

Yoga is an *analytical and visionary release* or, if we still believe in the language of doing or workout, it is at best VIVEKA WORKOUT (ever sifting Self from non-self).

Yoga Approaches

Yoga is holistic and embraces a wide range of approaches. Just imagine how comprehensive yoga is! It is empirical, rational, devotional, analytical, and philosophical. Yoga approaches, to our astonishment and delight, are perfectly compatible among themselves. Let us outline them a bit.

- **Samadhi** signifies *empirical* resolution (settlement) of mind through elaborate Ashtanga Yoga[7].

- The let-go approach called **Ishvara-pranidhana** (Surrender to God), which is part of Ashtanga Yoga, is *devotional* in character. It leads to perfection of Samadhi.

- If the above do not appeal to you, then Yoga persuades *rationally* and demonstrates **mind** (chitta) as intermediate and one not foolproof and ultimately reliable. … Prospective or retrospective – thinking can abstract one from actuality [here-now] to such an extent that one misses the available [present] and becomes unrealistic.[8] It therefore makes sense to quit thinking in far-fetched, fanciful, should-be, and regretful terms. … Relax thinking; be in yoga instantly. Do not fancy even benefits of yoga; experience them first-hand.

- In Yoga, **Purusha-khyati** is an *analytical* ongoing process of knowing or distinguishing Knower Self, by weaning off illusory non-self. Process itself is liberating and climaxes in knowledge of Self.

- Yoga is one of the six main orthodox philosophies of India. Its precise determination of **Avidya**[9] (Ignorance of Reality) remains unparalleled. The formula of wisdom provided by Yoga sheds light on the nature of things and transforms every misery into merit!

Yoga devotee can thus better appreciate other methods and have glimpse of the whole [*Brahma*]. … There indeed exist no approaches and ways such as non-yogic. All approaches fall within these broad categories.

---

[7] Ashtanga Yoga braces yoga devotee comprehensively.

[8] Absenting mentally and unawares is regarded as perversion in Yoga.

[9] Yoga proclaims Avidya as the root cause of all miseries (kleshas).

Viveka

VIVEKA[1] (Discrimination) [*Section 1*]
or Drashtri-Drishya Distinction[2]

in the backdrop of

peripheral **ASHTANGA YOGA** [*Section 2*]

and channelised through either or combinations of the following four:

MIND (chitta) [*Section 3*] unmasked as
medium, non-self, and conjurer

ISHVARA-PRANIDHANA (Surrender to God) [*Section 4*]
and demolishing myths of possession, choice, and doership (kartritva)

AVIDYA (Ignorance of Reality) [*Section 5*] identified as
the root cause of misery
that produces paradoxes of permanence, purity, pleasure (sukha), and personality [me-and-myness, or evanescent notions of self]

SELF (Atman) [*Section 6*] realised
as Purusha or Consciousness (Chiti) or Svartha (absolute existence)
and unlike paradoxical Drishya

metamorphoses into conviction of

KAIVALYA (intrinsic Liberation, or Establishment-in-Self)

FOOTNOTES

1. Samyoga and Avidya are not Viveka and therefore called *aviveka*. They produce pain (duhkha).
2. Complementary terms Drashtri (Seer/Knower) and Drishya (Seeable/Knowable) are intuitively coined as to signify Self and world, respectively. By virtue of its contrast to *Self*, the world can be called non-self (*other*).

Yoga jigsaw remains jumbled until the central, crucial piece Viveka is recovered. On its appreciation, things start falling in place. We sketched a bird's-eye view of the course that yoga can take within an individual. Here we got an opportunity to introduce key terms and ideas and their interrelationship in a flowchart fashion. Hopefully we have prepared a guide map for yoga trek!

This Book

Yoga jargon is daunting! Yoga sutras roughly 200 in number and those too in an ancient language could be too scary for the reader! That is the downside.

Nevertheless, there are good reasons for optimism. Firstly, the above outlines are sufficient to provide a ready reference. Secondly, the book is intended to provide a *Do It Yourself* liberating kit! It has used analysis to go beyond its confines [ANALYTICAL RELEASE]. It is not a scholarly work – if reader gets such an impression, I would not take it as a compliment. Thirdly, at the outset of the book is presented **SYNOPSIS** comprising eleven yoga sutras that are believed to provide mystic diagnosis and antidote. As the whole wisdom of yoga is stringed on sutras[10], so these handful sutras too retain the same insight and prove efficacious. Fulfilling experience and lifelong passion for yoga could be yours! Fourthly, there are introductory/preparatory messages opening sections and chapters. In addition, to make home the point, there are suggestive stories scattered throughout the book. Fifthly, Glossary of Sanskrit words [Appendix A] can prove handy for the reader. Sixthly, **TEACHER-DISCIPLE DIALOGUE** [Appendix B] contains excerpts from a work of the celebrated philosopher Shankara. It is remarkably precise, intuitive, and persuasive. I have personally used this dialogue as routine recitation. Lastly, original sources quoted in the book in support are expected to make reading an agreeable and engaging experience. Appendix C contains translation of all the yoga sutras. Yoga sutras in original, along with many other sources in Sanskrit, appear separately, at the end of the book [Appendix D].

---

[10] Sutra in Sanskrit means thread or string.

In this light, it is hoped that book brings home to the reader the mystery of uncanny passion for yoga!

Book preparation had been a solo affair. However, I sincerely appreciate whole-hearted faith and support of my wife (Shashi) – lack of which could have stunted my experiments!

This day, I (author) present the book to Trafford Publishing to make it available for readers worldwide – I appreciate their willingness and time-to-time guidance. The day is significant for two reasons: *Dussehra* festival of India – symbolic of triumph of good over evil; and Mahatma Gandhi's birth anniversary. I invite readers to have a look into the ancient wisdom presented in capsule form.

Hardev S. Thakur
at Manukau, NZ
the 2nd October, 2006

SYNOPSIS

DISEASE AND ANTIDOTE

☸

Mini yoga[11] worth reciting every morning

⁓ Diagnostic Sutras ⁓

- ❄ Illness (perceived or real), sloth, indecision, carelessness, laziness, obsessive indulgence/sensuality (literally, inability to withdraw), delusional thinking, Samadhi-not-attained (or instability), and Samadhi-not-maintained (or occasional stability): these nine *Mental Projections* are the obstacles (distractions) in the path of yoga. [I 30]

- ❄ Pain[12], rancour, physical restlessness [as in anxiety], and disturbed breathing [as in hyperventilation] accompany these Mental Projections. [I 31]

If any of these symptoms persists to disturb your calm, there is need for yoga discipline. To conquer these and to resolve mind, apply Antidote Sutras.

---

[11] Eleven sutras given here appear in original in Appendix D.

[12] It will be analysed in chapter 1.1.

Antidote Sutras

❄ Practise one principle. [I 32]

Living up to principles that you hold true is naturally agreeable. Look for and practise a principle that works in all situations.

Alternatively, ACCEPT ALL AS DIVINE as suggested in the holy phrase *Isha-vasya*[13]. World should be seen as pervaded by Lord [God Almighty]. ... Thence you own nothing and control nothing! You realise yourself a true servant, trustee, and custodian; and escape blame and sin!

BE FAIR TO ALL, as you would like it to yourself. [BG VI 31-32]. To discriminate or be unfair to anyone is not only unlawful[14] but sinful as well.

BE TRUE TO ONENESS. Practise Yamas and Niyamas [*see* chapters 2.2 and 2.3] *but not selectively.*

As animal is to men, so is *violator of oneness* to gods – thus runs the ultimate admonition [*see* chapter 6.4].

❄ **Friendliness** toward happy and fortunate people, instead of jealousy and envy; **compassion** toward unhappy and unfortunate, instead of apathy and fault-finding; **willing cooperation** with righteous and pious, instead of deserting and purging them; and **indifference** (non-cooperation) toward wicked, instead of helping and approving their acts — cultivation of such attitudes restores cheerfulness; [I 33]

---

13 On the contrary, anīśvara (no-lord) is a self-doubting, fatalistic, and anarchic attitude.

14 Fairness is what justice really is. (Justice Potter Stewart)

❄ Ejecting breath and holding it out [and repeating it several times] too brightens mood; [I 34]

[*See* Pranayama in chapter 2.4 to find the manner of holding breath out using fingers.]

Its benefits are amazing! We know at times we become crazy about things in life and which we regret later. However, this technique produces instant foresight and withdrawal.

❄ Alternatively, consciously absorb (engage) in activities and thoughts, and settle mind; [I 35]

Simply said, work while you work; play while you play. Be MENTALLY PRESENT. Attention on physical and mental objects/activities steadies the mind. *Know* what you are knowing or doing.

Unfortunately, we are in the habit of doing and knowing unconsciously (*i.e.*, unknowingly or out of ignorance). We thereby conform (identify with) activities and mental processes (in other words, mind) and overlook the distinction. To break this habit, first be aware of non-routine physical activities, then of every physical activity, later of mental processes (thought, memory, delusion, etc.), and lastly of every mental process.

In metaphysical terminology, with attentive (*sattva*) physical activity (*rajas*), you overcome *tamas* (inertia, depression, insanity, and ignorance) and become aware of inner radiance to be mentioned next. ... *Attentive* actions are a precursor of Karma Yoga.[15]

---

[15] Perfection in Karma Yoga comes with the Yoga of Knowledge (jñāna yoga) [*i.e.*, with the knowledge of Self or when the illusion of selish works recedes].

❄ Or be aware of sorrowless[16], absolute inner-radiance[17] (Consciousness); [I 36]

See chapter 6.2 where meditation on Yoga phrase *for the sake of Self* (svartha) is suggested.[18]

❄ Or attune to, esteem, or live in the company of, someone wise who has humbled attachment, greed, and selfishness and for whom no purpose of life remains to be fulfilled[19]; [I 37]

❄ Or keep dream and sleep in perspective – deliberate and question the verity of waking life; [I 38]

In waking, dream, and deep sleep states, experiences of one state are negated in others. [*See* chapters 6.2 and 6.3.]

Moreover, with passage of time, waking life looks like dream!

'All that we see or seem
Is but a dream within a dream.' (Edgar Allan Poe)

---

16 All sorrows and delusions stem from other (non-self, drishya/*seeable*) and never from Self (Consciousness, Drashtri/*Seer*).

17 Imagine that Sun is not there (as at night), nor Moon (as in moonless night). There is no fire (light) too, nor voice (to illumine/guide you where is what). Despite such terrible darkness, can you deny *light within* (consciousness)? Don't you know which one your right hand is? … You *are* self-luminous – this light requires no material fuel and wick! Note the names like स्वयंज्योतिःपुरुष (svayañjyoṭiḥ puruṣa) and हिरण्यगर्भ (hiraṇyagarbha, golden embryo).

18 स्वार्थसंयमात् पुरुषज्ञानम्। (svārṭhasaṃyamāṭ puruṣajñānam.) [III 35]

19 puruṣārṭhaśūnya [IV 34]

❄ Alternatively, *contemplate* whatever you will or appeals to you. [I 39]

However, be aware of your absorption; avoid stupor.

❄ Comprehend Avidya (Ignorance of Reality) as misjudgement of impermanent, impure (elusive), pain, and non-self as their opposites. [II 5]

Here Yoga provides a succinct checklist of wisdom. Eschew paradoxes of permanence, purity, pleasure, and personality [me-and-myness; evanescent notions of Self], wherein lies potential Avidya [*see* section 5].

✵

SECTION ONE

Yoga Vision

VIVEKA

Knower (Self) is distinct from known or knowable.

DRASHTRI-DRISHYA DISTINCTION

CHAPTERS

Aviveka is haven for troubles.[20] [*Sanskrit proverb*]

In Yoga, Aviveka (indiscrimination) means:

1) *Samyoga* (knowledge contrary to Viveka) and
2) *Avidya* (Ignorance of Reality).

---

[20] अविवेकः परमापदां पदम्। (avivekaḥ paramāpadām padam.)

CHAPTER ONE

Confuse Self and Suffer

Other names used for Self are Atman/Atma, Purusha, Drashtri (literally, Seer), Consciousness, Awareness, and Witness. The Bhagavad Gita suggestively uses Me and I. UNCLUTTER THE CONFUSION; CONCENTRATE ON TWO CATEGORIES: *DRASHTRI* AND *DRISHYA*. ...

So don't I know who I am? For example, I am conscious. I know. At least I am Knower (Drashtri). ... Unfortunately, that is not the end!

In our notion of Self get mixed many objects or thought objects which are either known or knowable (*i.e.*, drishya; seeable). Alternatively, we identify ourselves with objects that are non-self; we overlook the distinction (Viveka). In Yoga, we call it as Drashtri obscured by Drishya.

Yoga does not regard this error innocent and forgivable. Thence, out of compassion, Yoga admonishes:

Samyoga (or Drashtri-Drishya Conjunction) is the cause (hetu) of pain (heya). It is caused by Avidya. [II 17, 24]

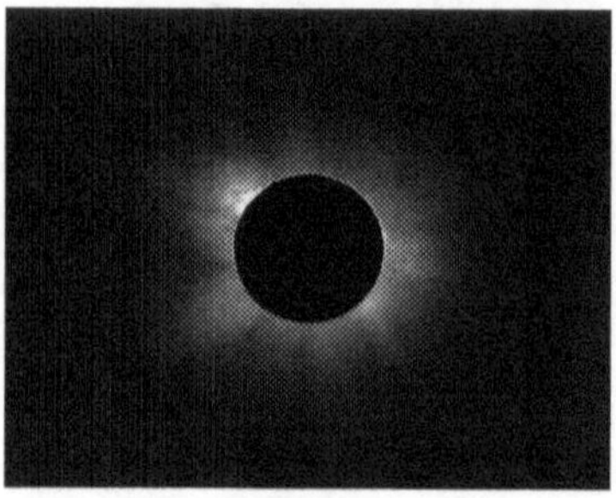

Samyoga can be called as ECLIPSE OF SELF (DRASHTRI/SEER) by world (Drishya/Seeable).

To confuse true Self with non-self is to suffer. Forgetting and confusing Self with world (*other*) are suggestively conveyed in this old parable.

Once there lived ten worldly-wise [or *other*wise[21]] men who set off to some town to earn money for themselves. On the way, they had to cross a rivulet. They crossed it but suspiciously. On reaching the other side, they thought it appropriate to count themselves in order to be sure about their number. They were horrified to find one of them missing. Each one counted others severally and each time the count did not go beyond nine. It was even more embarrassing for them when they were unable to recollect who the missing one was! ... Each one of them was so lost in others as to ignore oneself.

In Zen, situation is described as 'host lost in guests.'

---

[21] Other is indicative of non-self.

Yoga and yoga

Yoga Sutras of Patanjali is an ancient Sanskrit text comprising 195 sutras[22] on yoga written by Sage Patanjali. In short, we use the word Yoga for this source book; and the word yoga for discipline and philosophy that go by this name. The book Yoga embodies Vedic philosophy and historically dates back to 2nd century B.C. This in fact is a codification of an elaborate, then-prevailing customary system. Possibly, yoga is very ancient!

Yoga sutras are divided into four chapters (also called quarters), namely: Samadhi (the first quarter), Means (Sadhana, the second), Glory (Vibhuti, the third quarter), and Kaivalya (the fourth). With Yoga stands associated the commentary of Sage Vyasa on sutras – that is the earliest and highly relied commentary.

Yoga is popular as a physical discipline. However, it is philosophy as well that delivers. Rather, the only practical, dynamic philosophy helps us overcome physical and psychological odds comprehensively and establishes us in philosophy-free state!

It is appropriate to first outline the purport and scheme of Yoga. The purport remains general in nature and is typical of an ideal philosophy; and scheme unique and realistic. These are set out in Quarter II *Means* of Yoga, more particularly sutras 12-28. As medical science attempts to determine four types of issues: disease, cause of disease, health, and means of health, so too Yoga proceeds to determine pain (heya), cause of pain (heya-hetu), Escape or Kaivalya (hana), and means of Escape/Kaivalya (hana-upaya).

Rest of the chapter is devoted to explain these.

---

[22] In Sanskrit, sutra means aphorism or threadlike proposition.

Pain (*Heya*)

The very objective of yoga is to overcome, or escape, pain (duhkha). According to Yoga, pain is heya (meaning worth-escaping or what-is-to-be-escaped). This heya (pain) would be acceptable for targeting even from the standpoint of a layperson. Who doesn't want to get rid of pain!

This is not all. Yoga is the only philosophy that targets pain in totality: physical as well as mental. ... This makes yoga a comprehensive and most relevant philosophy for us who are constantly afflicted by the paradox of pleasure.

But, what about the vivekin (one who exercises Viveka, or discriminates between Self and non-self)? It is no different for him. This entire world is pain for him too – thus postulates Yoga the universality of pain. Yoga elucidates its wide incidence by pointing to its varieties such as: end-result pain, instant pain, chain of pain (in the form of samskaras). Yoga explains the metaphysical and perceptional basis of pain too.

- The pain-in-the-end includes those experiences that are pleasant while experienced, but ultimately, over time result in pain. For example, hedonistic and wanton life results in physical drain, and gives rise to chain of bad habits such as rash desire, anger, attachment (and greed), and aversion (hatred). Therefore, what meets the eye may not be pleasure!
- Next comes instantaneous pain as in sensations of burn. Unexpected events, reckless acts, and irrational thinking (such as feelings of envy) produce anguish and instant pain. Uncertainty – unpredictable change whether actual, potential, or perceived – shrouds every aspect of life and creates a sense of insecurity and fear.

- ❄ Chain of pain stems from habits or samskaras[23] (impressions) that yield intermittent pain, even in distant future and unseen lives. These impressions finding suitable occasion become active and influence our intentions, leading to fixed, habitual behaviour and result patterns. According to Yoga, samskaras form a crucial link in the misery-generating Klesha-chain[24]. This chain manifests itself in train of births, life spans, and experiences.
- ❄ There are three metaphysical constituents (*gunas*) of Nature (*Prakriti*). World is regarded as a modification (vikriti) of these elemental gunas. Their names solve the mystery of disturbance, conflict, and pain of world. They are ***sattva*** (light, knowledge), ***rajas*** (greed, motion, activity), and ***tamas*** (mass, inertia, ignorance). In terms of modern physics, world is a play of light, motion, and mass (matter). In spiritual terms, **1)** knowledge and ignorance remain contrary; **2)** all activities are ultimately instigated by a mixture of ignorance and not by pure knowledge; and **3)** rajas keeps us impatient and restless. ... Their (gunas') different proportions at different times produce difference/conflict/restlessness in moods, intentions, and personalities!
- ❄ Pain can also be traced to our *wishful* and *expectant* thinking, that is somewhat random, arbitrary, and at variance with actuality (here-now).
- ❄ Pleasure and pain (being dependent on our interpretation and perspective) have to be transferable, alternating experiences. ... Or pleasure is transitory and is ultimately pain.
- ❄ Drishya (world), being non-self (other), explains the universality of pain. Because of distinction (Viveka), it is not feasible to bridge to worldly pleasures!

---

[23] They are memories only but separated in time or place or by births. [IV 9]

[24] *Kleshas* (the Miseries), *karmas* (actions), *phalas* (fruits/results), and *samskaras* together form this vicious, self-feeding chain.

- Avidya[25] instigates all our actions and thought processes. Results will eventually be painful.

Every experience is another name for pain! [Explanations will keep coming up throughout the book.]

---

[25] Avidya is described as Klesha (misery), rather the root Klesha.

Cause of Pain (*Samyoga*)

Next comes investigation into cause of pain, called in Yoga as heya-hetu. As already stated in the introduction to chapter, pain is caused by **Drashtri-Drishya Conjunction**, which has its roots in Avidya (ignorance). ...

It is natural to suspect bias and pessimism in the statement 'the entire world is indeed pain.' Can't cause of pain be plainly demonstrated like light and darkness? ... Yes, it can be.

For that, we first need to understand the terms Drashtri and Drishya.

The words Drashtri and Drishya are derived from a common verb in the sense 'to see (or know).' ... In Yoga, accordingly, **Drashtri** means Seer, Knower, or Consciousness. [II 20]

Likewise, Drishya means worth-seeing or seeable[26] [or worth-knowing or knowable] – whatever that can be perceived and conceived. ... However, in Yoga the term is described as world along with its material and efficient cause (Prakriti).[27] ... It therefore is reasonable here to take **Drishya** in both senses: seeable (knowable) and world.

Drashtri (knower) and Drishya (knowable) are distinct and mutually exclusive, but together all-inclusive. ... Understandably, Drashtri, being undeniable, subsists as true ***Self***; and Drishya is fit to be regarded as non-self (or ***other***), in conformity with Viveka.

---

[26] Though seeable is a non-standard word, but it conveys the sense exactly.

[27] Drishya is described as play or modification of three gunas (*i.e.*, sattva, rajas, and tamas); assuming forms of gross elements, senses, and self [ego or personality]; and providing experience (bhoga) to ignorant and liberation to enlightened. [II 18]

Accordingly, it needs to be remembered that WHATEVER I CAN PERCEIVE OR CONCEIVE IS NON-SELF (NOT ME). Mindfulness of this axiomatic distinction is **Viveka** (विवेक); and its oversight **Samyoga** (संयोग, cause of pain).

Yoga further reveals: Drishya exists for the sake of or by virtue of Drashtri. [II 21] … [We shall build up on these threads later.]

This Drashtri-Drishya distinction is plain and lucid compared to similar but cryptic Sattva-Purusha distinction.

Our pain lies in Samyoga (*i.e.,* in oversight or obscuration of *essential* distinction between Drashtri and Drishya). Samyoga deludes in the form of identifications with Drishya. In the process, characteristics of Drishya like change and becoming are superimposed on changeless[28] and pure[29] Drashtri. Here are a few illustrations:

- What happens when we see from a close distance a river with strong current? We are whirled! Isn't it a sensation? Or is it actual?
- What happens at the loss of *my* possessions (which are objects of knowledge, or Drishya)? *I* (pseudo possessor) feel myself lost! Isn't self-loss false?
- *My* objects, organs, and feelings seem to define *me* (Drashtri)! They indeed create my personality and not me!
- Situations *themselves* undergo change but, surprisingly, those move *me* and perturb *me*. Really?

In Samyoga, world (other/non-self) affects, superimposes on, and appears as, Self. Samyoga (oversight of essential distinction) therefore has rightly been postulated as pain.

Water assumes shapes and colours of containers, though in reality it is formless, undivided, and neutral. Drashtri too is neutral

---

[28] YS IV 18

[29] YS II 20

(pure), undivided, and changeless, but is identified with and affected by body, senses, and mind. Furthermore, as water is different from reflections on its surface and from objects reflected on it, so is Drashtri (Self) different from mental reflections (thoughts, memories, delusions, and knowledge) and from objects of thought.

However, by oversight of distinction, *pure* Drashtri is mistakenly seen as tainted by sin. By same oversight, *just knowing* Drashtri is mistakenly seen as sometimes happy, sometimes sad; sometimes enriched, sometimes ripped.

The Upanishads establish this distinction through the admonition *'not this, not this'* (NETI NETI). The admonition signifies that Drashtri (Self) is neither this nor that. Self is distinct from *changing* world (Drishya). ... [In a sense, Self is also established as unchanging and unruffled!]

Escape (*Kaivalya*) and its Means (*Viveka*)

Now it is quite natural to expect Yoga to discuss Escape (hana) and Means of Escape (hana-upaya). As natural corollary to the discussion so far, Escape should happen the moment Avidya or Samyoga ceases. Equivalently, Escape is accomplished through ceaseless display of Viveka (or no longer confusion of Self). Sage Vyasa calls Viveka as Right Vision (samyak darshana).

The state realised through Viveka is **Kaivalya** (कैवल्य; literally, aloneness) – that is free from plaintive desire for company and possessions. Self is liberated from the woes of world (*other*). Simple reason is that It is not confused and identified with the world.

Yoga describes this liberated state (Kaivalya) in a more insightful way. It calls it *establishment in one's own nature or self.*[30] ... This description is placed in the beginning and again at the conclusion of yoga sutras; this bespeaks its eminence among key terms of Yoga!

Hence, action, effort, becoming, or seeking fulfilment outside or at some future point ought not to be compatible with yoga. Yoga is not to be achieved at some future point of time. [See Diagnostic Sutras of Synopsis.] It is simply ESTABLISHMENT-IN-SELF (BEING NATURAL SELF).

Lastly, let us make a passing mention of how **discriminative knowledge** (knowledge born of Viveka) can be distinguished.

This knowledge is intuitive and transcendent and still comprehensive and directable at all objects and in all conditions. It is unlike customary knowledge that is piecemeal and progressive (gained in stages or degrees) and is based on authorities and

---

30 स्वरूपेऽवस्थानम् (svarūpe'vasṭhānam) [I 3] and स्वरूपप्रतिष्ठा (svarūpa-praṭiṣthā) [IV 34]

inference [I 48-49, III 54]. This knowledge is objective (here-now).

Man of Viveka (vivekin) lives in the present moment and remains objective (here-and-now) and realistic (relevant to all times) whereas others struggle to adapt themselves to changing times. [*Cf.* III 52.] ... Obsession with future and past is a mental disease!

To ensure Viveka, one needs to be ever wary and critical.

SEEING IS NOT BELIEVING HERE.

Isn't it paradoxical? [For us, seeing is believing.][31] Whatever you see is not you! Moreover, it may not exist the way you see! Or it may not exist at all!

---

31 चक्षुर्वै ब्रह्म। (chakṣurvāi brahma) [BU IV i 4] 'This eye is verily Brahma.' What it sees is believed to exist!

CHAPTER TWO

Effortless, Analytical Yoga

Now we proceed to scan textual evidence as to clear any misgivings about yoga.

> As Avidya (Ignorance of Reality) ceases, so does Samyoga — this is **Escape**, or **Kaivalya** (Liberation) of Drashtri (Self) from painful world.
>
> Escape is accomplished through undisturbed display/practice of **Viveka** (Discrimination).
>
> *Yoga Sutras II 25-26*

Does 'Escape' of last chapter sound life-negative or life-evasive? It is not so indeed. It is participative and full of life. Any such suspicion stands resolved in view of mention in Yoga *viz.* 'actions of yogi as neither moral nor immoral, unlike those of common people.' [IV 7] …

There can be another doubt! How can we be active and extrovert and still effortless and our natural selves? … Unfortunately, this doubt draws support from Yoga text. For example, Yoga calls itself *discipline*. [I 1] [The word discipline sounds physical, earthly.] … Similarly, Yoga has prescribed a *practical path to yoga* [II 1] and, in addition, calls its second chapter as *Means*. Moreover, Ashtanga Yoga, which includes physical postures and exercises, has been dealt at length in Yoga – roughly thirty sutras spanning two chapters (Means and Glory) are devoted to this purpose. ...

Odds prevail in favour of treating yoga as physical, extrovert, and practical discipline only! But how long! ... Precisely, word used in original for discipline means 'subsequent authority or ruling' or 'exposition of already-prevailing authority.'

Escape of Yoga remains effortless, abstract, and analytical. Isn't it evident from introductory sutras where it is said: 'as ignorance ceases' and 'through Viveka'[32]?

Ideally, Yoga is innate and intrinsic. It is not a consequence or effect of arrangements and practices. This is evident from Yoga itself such as:

- 'Yoga is *Samadhi* and it is the *nature* (*dharma*) of mind in *all* the five mental states.'[33]
- Yoga is *not union or unification* – so clarifies the commentator Vachaspati Mishra[34]. Uniting predicates duality, activity, effort, and temporal limitation. For instance, union of two will be achieved with effort and activity at some future point of time. Then union is bound to break up sometime!
- In the last chapter, Viveka was called as Right Vision. Let us see what Sage Vyasa has to advise about that:

> Right Vision (Viveka) is free from literal improvements or eliminations (strippings) in Self. If we accept improvements in Self, then Self is the effect (result) of causes, and any such improvement is transitory, short-lived! Similarly, if we accept eliminations, that also goes against immutability of Self.

Hence, yoga does not stand for literal acquisition or

---

32 That is, through distinguishing Self from non-self

33 Sage Vyasa's comment on YS I 1

34 vāchaspaṭi miśra

deliverance.

- Yoga is defined as inhibition (nirodha) of mental processes. [I 2] The two words 'nirodha' and 'mental' decisively dispel any misgivings about yoga. The term nirodha in Yoga means *'detachment practised over time.'* [I 12] ... Together they suggest that life of yoga is unlike life driven by impulses, emotions, and selfish motives! Moreover, yoga targets mind because *mind is subtle, close (intimate), and initiator*[35] in relation to outer and adherent physical body. ... Therefore, physical workouts and practices remain incidental and circumferential. Any action-based approach prescribed by Yoga can be expedient but remains superficial in deed as far as essential yoga is concerned.

- Yoga extols **Knowledge of Self** in such words as Purusha-khyati. [I 16] When Self is realised (recognised), there naturally follows enduring and genuine detachment ('superior detachment') that in turn leads to ultimate *non-cognitive Samadhi*. [I 18] ... Our pursuits like games of childhood become meaningless and themselves get dropped painlessly as we mature and seek for or realise the superior [Self]. [*Cf.* BG II 59.] ... Of course, realisation of Self is cerebral and therefore *effort*less! Yoga therefore cannot be effected or brought about in material sense.

- Moreover, how can actions and practices – being temporal and limited – be expected to produce an eternal life hereafter?

- What we call 'failure in attaining Samadhi' and 'failure in retaining Samadhi' are not actual failures. They are product of distorted thinking. By calling such failures as **mental projections**, Yoga questions their appropriateness and nips irrational thinking well in advance. [I 30]

---

[35] No physical violence is violence unless it is intentional or it primarily serves some selfish motive. [*Cf.* BG XVIII 17.] Unintended violence is an innocent accident. On the other hand, an intentional violent attempt – which may not have harmed any body – is fit to be regarded as wrongdoing.

- *Surrender to God* is Yoga's favourite approach. It is direct in accomplishing Samadhi. [II 45] ... **Surrender** is neither an activity nor voluntary! [We shall revert to it in section 4.]

- Let us now consider Ashtanga Yoga. Word *ashtanga* literally means eight-limbed. So Ashtanga Yoga should not be confused as eight-staged or eight-stepped.[36] Further, according to Yoga, all yoga limbs (including Samadhi) are *outer and peripheral* from vantage point.[37] [III 7-8] ... On realisation, all practices prove to be incidental and not fundamental.

Let us recapitulate. Escape or yoga is not life evasive. It rather embraces life with Right Vision (Viveka).

Escape or Kaivalya (Liberation) dawns with Viveka (Discrimination), or with the cessation of Avidya. In Viveka, one repudiates observable world (Drishya). ... But if one continues to identify with, crave for, and favour or victimise, some/part, his conduct is repugnant to Viveka.

Viveka does not involve physical effort. It is simply Right Vision. ... However, in its absence, life is nightmare! In ignorance of Self, one is not even truly selfish! Sincere objectives of self-fulfilment too will lead one astray! [38] ... Without Right Vision, we live in ignorance and lead others too into ignorance, like blind man leading other blinds. [KU II 5]

---

[36] Yoga has used word bhūmi for stage or state. The word aňga means limb.

[37] First two limbs (yama and niyama) appear to be crucial building blocks of yoga; rest of limbs are sequels. For instance, yamas are mandatory principles. [II 31] Among niyamas (personal rules), last three are revered as 'practical path to yoga.' [II 1] The last niyama, Surrender to God (Ishvara-pranidhana) directly leads to Samadhi. [II 45] Third and fourth limbs (asana and pranayama) expedite physico-psychological fitness and break habitual and obsessive mental behaviour (or divert mind).

[38] If you donot know where you are going, every road will get you nowhere. (Henry Kissinger)

Yoga is effortless, analytical liberation. Effortlessness, of course, is achieved without effort! ... Yoga is just being our natural selves (or establishment in Self), unlike doing and becoming. It looks incredible! But for how long!

Ashtanga Yoga that is taken up in the next section provides substructure for making yoga a reality and Viveka a conviction. We shall expand on Samyoga (the cause of pain) in later sections, *e.g.*, in *Mind* as our identifications with mind and its processes; in *Surrender to God* as choice, possessions, and doership (false agency); and in sections *Avidya* and *Self* as ignorance of Reality and Self, respectively.

SECTION TWO

Ashtanga Yoga

EIGHT-LIMBED YOGA

YOGA IN PRACTICE

CHAPTERS

Tiny ripples of Viveka can produce colossal waves in distant shores of time and are capable of purging our judgement of biases and prejudices. Seeing is not simply believing – no belief is left unexamined[39].

[This conscious questioning[40] is godsend. This will repudiate inessential within and establish us in true Self!]

[39] Unexamined life is not worth living. (Socrates)

[40] It refers to Viveka.

Over time then...

what we see is *virtual* rather than actual;

a *concept* instead of entity;

a *dream* and not reality! ...

Seemingly

doing,

thinking,

moving[41] ...

What we called objective is *subjective.*

Yoga is a *realisation* rather than attainment;

involuntary instead of volitional!

41 ध्यायतीव लेलायतीव। (ḍhyāyaṭīva lelāyaṭīva) [BU IV iii 7]

CHAPTER ONE

Overview

❋

In this paradoxical background, it will be easier to appreciate the essential nature of yoga and its morality. Yoga is intrinsic and not an accessory!

Ashtanga Yoga as its name in Sanskrit suggests has eight limbs and ideally climaxes in the conviction of Viveka. [II 28] The limbs are:

- ❋ **Yamas** (Laws of Life) – five social obligations
- ❋ **Niyamas** (Rules) – five personal obligations
- ❋ **Asana** (Physical Posture)
- ❋ **Pranayama** (Life-expansive Energy/Breathing)
- ❋ **Pratyahara** (Withdrawal of Senses)
- ❋ **Dharana** (Concentration)
- ❋ **Dhyana** (Contemplation)
- ❋ **Samadhi** (Meditation)

CHAPTER TWO

Yamas

❄

PRINCIPLES THAT REDEEM

अहिंसा
Ahimsa
(Non-violence)

सत्य
Satya
(Truthfulness, Integrity)

अस्तेय
Asteya
(Non-stealing, Honesty)

ब्रह्मचर्य
Brahmacharya
(Devout Life)

अपरिग्रह
Aparigraha
(Non-covetousness)

In Yoga, these are the five laws regarded **mandatory** and **indispensable**. They together constitute an august vow that is not to be compromised by anyone anywhere and in any circumstance. [II 31] These laws form the very basis of yoga. These are obligatory on yoga devotee during initial stages; but, later, for the realised one, these become conviction.

Ahimsa (Non-violence)

This law forbids intentional harm to life in any form (especially for personal or selfish reasons). This ruling on non-harming of life is absolute. Yoga is categorical in its disapproval of violence:

> Ill will, violence, or similar anti-life (anti-God) intentions and practices are prompted by greed, anger, and delusion; and are accompanied with endless pain and ignorance. It does not matter whether these practices are carried out personally [done], caused through others [abetted], or approved in others [condoned]. [II 34]

COUNTER WHY WITH WHY-NOT. Warning: if you relax principle partly, you end up relaxing it totally!

One may wrongly reason in favour of violence, saying, 'Self is said to be immortal and bodies are mortal – so what harm!' Such argument is immature and erroneous. The very advocates of violence would not accept it and call it foul when they themselves are vulnerable or victims.

Similarly, one may detract devotees by such arguments as: Ahimsa is unachievable or unavoidable. But remember: Ahimsa is mandatory. ... Violence is not the rule but exception – just like in a civilised society, capital punishment is not the rule but exception.

Once in my city (Manukau, Auckland), I happened to see a jeep that displayed a message at its rear. It was an inspiring appeal enclosed between Om symbols.

ॐ BE KIND TO ANIMALS. DO NOT KILL THEM. ॐ

I was impressed by the compassion of the sponsor. ... We should not forget that kindness begets kindness. ... Alas! Generally, taste dictates, not compassion.

Ahimsa and other Yamas should ever remain our guiding principles.

OUR FOOD SHOULD BE VEGETARIAN. There are good arguments[42] in favour of vegetarian diet, like:

- *Human intestines* differ in structure from those of carnivores. They are long and pocketed; and are thus well suited for vegetarian food.
- We need sufficient dietary *fibre* (also called roughage) in our daily food. Luckily, vegetarian food consisting of whole grains, vegetables, fruits, and nuts has it in abundance. Fibre in food helps in removing toxic materials from our intestines.
- When we eat meat, we obtain *third-hand energy*.[43] Vegetarian food provides second-hand energy – it is therefore less wasteful.
- We feed animals in order to feed meat eaters. However, data show that it is more *expensive* than feeding people directly.
- There are environmental costs too. Every year we lose more forests. Forests are cut down and turned into grazing fields for animals.
- Fear and pain of subject animals sneak into meat eaters and make them *emotionally vulnerable*. This perhaps explains for increase in number of psychotic conditions!

Alas! Generally, taste dictates, not reason and facts.

I am reminded of a parable from The Puranas (source books on Hindu mythology) about goddess Parvati. [Myths are relevant for all times. They leave an enduring message on faithful audience.] The goddess had led a very

---

[42] These arguments appear in detail in the book *YOGA Mind & Body* of Sivananda Yoga Vedanta Centre.

[43] Sun is the primary source of energy. Plants are secondary.

austere life in order to realise Lord Shiva [Reality[44]]. ... To that end, she observed such an exemplary Ahimsa that she ate only those fruits which themselves had dropped off the trees. At that point, her kinsfolk called out in awe, 'U ma!' (Leave it; enough of it!) ... She did not yield to counter arguments and succeeded in her objective. ... She then onward was known in the worlds by the name Uma[45]. ...

---

[44] saṭyam-śivam-sunḍaram (सत्यं शिवं सुन्दरम्।) Truth is beneficial and beautiful! False is elusive.

[45] umā

Satya (Truthfulness, Integrity)

My father once finding me upset [I am grateful to that occasion!] told me an anecdote of Kuru princes of The Mahabharata epic. The princes were sent to guru (teacher) Drona for initiation into learning, archery, and warfare. The first day the topic taken up by the teacher was 'anger.' He explained to them anger and its demerits with simple stories. Next day, before taking up the next lesson, teacher wanted to check whether students had grasped their lesson well. Many of them showed confidence to reproduce it on asking. Some confessed their inability! The teacher did not expect this from well-groomed princes. He showed his annoyance and warned them to rehearse it well by next day without fail.

The third day teacher anxiously enquired the same from princes. Now Yudhishthira was the only one who still had not learnt. Teacher could no more help chastising such waywardness and gave him a smack. It was disappointing for teacher. ... But it bewildered him too when Yudhishthira in no time admitted, 'I have learnt the lesson now!'

When asked about this instant turnabout, Yudhishthira explained, 'This time, anger did not surface within me, even when smacked; so I have now learnt (*practised*) the lesson.' ...

This is truthfulness: sincere application in life of what we hold true and abstain from what we ideally do not approve. Otherwise, there is hypocritical respect for principles. Without Satya, life becomes sham. ...

In Sanskrit, words sat (सत्) and satya (सत्य) do not mean the same. Sat connotes truth, reality, existence; and satya *worth-existing* or *ideal* (TRUTH IN PRINCIPLE). For example, if sat is true (as opposed to false), satya is for moral, reasonable, or right (as opposed to wrong). ...

The word satya is a logical necessity because we do not see truth or reality (sat) *as it is;* we see truth *as perceived by us.* There can be difference between *ideal* [should be] and *actual* [is]!

Therefore, the principle Satya enjoins PRACTICE AND PROFESSION OF 'TRUTH IN PRINCIPLE'. It is *integrity* – CONSISTENCY IN THOUGHT, EXPRESSION, AND ACTION. This is Truthfulness.

Truthfulness is *never inopportune.* It is never too late to begin and there is no reason for letup. This is a serious advice because we unwittingly slip! We believe in something else, say something else, and still do something quite contrary. For example, we profess the benefits of meat eating, but hardly do we confess that largely it is the taste, that compels us to speak in favour of it. …

Truthfulness will ultimately provide opportunities for transparent discussions, tangible results, and resolution of conflicts.

Asteya (Non-stealing, Honesty)

In Sanskrit, it literally means NOT WORTH STEALING. Yoga regards nothing in this world worth stealing – *the most valuable lies within. ...*

The term Asteya signifies the value honesty — NEITHER ACQUIRING ANYTHING NOR DENYING ANYONE, UNDULY AND UNFAIRLY. It could be that we do not harm any body and thus believe that we do not violate Ahimsa principle, but we still could be cheating others. Similarly, while observing Satya principle, we may be true to ourselves [doing what we hold true], but we may not be true to society. Hence the necessity of this law Asteya.

Accordingly, dishonesty, misappropriation, tax evasion, etc. ought to be desisted. Keep watch over *ignorant* and *greedy* motives behind!

I remember one incident of my childhood. One day while I was studying, my fountain pen ran out of ink. I had no ink with me to fill in. There was office on the ground floor of the building – my father used to be in charge of that. I went to the office and told the people there [my father was not there; he was on tour] that I needed ink to fill my pen. I was offered a big bottle containing around 1 litre of ink and was advised that I should get an empty bottle from home to get some supply of ink. It sounded great!

I came back home. I wrote with the pen and even found the writing in royal blue ink very impressive. I shared the whole incident with my father on his return from tour. He simply advised me to buy my own ink! ...

Yes, given limited resources, we are obliged to draw a line between what is legitimately ours and what is not ours. We need to exercise discretion every moment.

Brahmacharya (Devout Life)

It is mistakenly interpreted as celibacy alone.

Precisely, it signifies the life of devout pupil – dedicated to study of The Vedas and to service of Boundless Being/God in all. This is the meaning of word Brahma/ Brahman.

Therefore, Brahmacharya can be carried on even beyond pupil stage, into later life stages or roles, namely: those of householder, recluse, and hermit. It does not conflict with any stage.

Devotee practises broadmindedness, continence, and chastity; studies scriptures; and watches against (and rids himself of) obsession, greed, fear, and perturbation.

Aparigraha (Non-covetousness)

In terms of Viveka, objects remain distinct and therefore ungraspable. ... Greedy hoarding is depraving!

Keep wants to prudent minimum and use resources scrupulously. This will save resources for the community and eliminate shortages from world. ... Without this principle, we would tend to be extravagant and oblivious of the needs of others, to the point of 'harming life.'

My father used to take personal care of the enlightened saint of his village. One day he was washing his clothes and gave them a final, firm wring. That alerted the saint who was watching all this. The saint advised him not to do so (as to weaken the texture of clothes) – no matter if clothes would dry in a little longer time. ...

I remember another time when my father had left for heavens. I with my mother was returning from Haridwar after immersing his ashes in the Ganges, holy river. We had to catch a late night train. On the railway platform, we had dinner in the railway canteen. After the meal, I got up to move, but my mother was busy in wrapping leftover rotis (loaves of bread). To me it did not look dignifying! ... She *corrected* me, saying 'Is it wise to let food [which gives life to us] be thrown to bin or drain?' ...

These five Yamas lay the foundation of yoga. One should not even think of deviating form these. If there are allurements and temptations against these, contemplate the counter arguments already stated. [II 34]

FOOD CONTENT

With due deference to Yamas, our food should not constitute harm to life, nor cheating, nor denial of due share to others. Food can be divided into three categories (corresponding to dominating guna), namely: sattva-rich (vitalising), rajas-rich (stimulating), and tamas-rich (depressing).

Whole grains, fruits, vegetables, legumes, nuts, honey, milk, butter, etc. are rich in **sattva** (vitality). They are naturally delicious and satisfying – one cannot be greedy or obsessed about these! Take care as not to debase their quality. Eggs, meat, poultry, and fish are taboo. ... Prefer roughage (fibre); avoid fat.

When food is artificially sweetened and flavoured or is too salty, fatty, pungent, spicy, or fried, it becomes **rajas** in quality (or mood enhancer). It can overstimulate and cause restlessness and discontent in us. Tea, coffee, and caffeinated drinks also fall into this category.

Rotten, stale, fermented (e.g., alcoholic drinks), processed, and preserved foods are **tamas**-rich. These produce gloom, stupor, and depression.

According to Yoga, benefits of Yamas accrue to devotee, like: hostilities disappear around him; his actions bear fruits; riches draw in to him; he gains potency; and he understands wherefore [purpose] of life, respectively. ...

But benefit at the level of society could be ... WHOLESALE REDEMPTION with social justice and order in a worthy and meritorious way. Every being secures fair share of resources and ensures the same for all. ...

Yoga is a beginning, not an end. Carefully avoid complacency about Yamas and Niyamas – these require to be ever pursued sincerely.

CHAPTER THREE

Niyamas

❋

PRACTICAL PATH TO YOGA

शौच
Shaucha
(Cleanliness)

सन्तोष
Santosha
(Contentment)

तपः
Tapas
(Endurance)

स्वाध्याय
Svadhyaya
(Study of Self)

ईश्वरप्रणिधान
Ishvara-pranidhana
(Surrender to God)

In Yoga, these are the five rules for observance by everyone. These reflect obligations more as to oneself.

Shaucha (Cleanliness)

It stands for physical hygiene and cleanliness. In spiritual terms, it signifies moral and pure intentions and conduct.[46]

Its perfection is stated to produce effects like disillusionment with physical body [own as well as others']; intentional purity; cheerfulness; one-pointedness [Samadhi!]; mastery of senses; and fitness for realisation of Self. [II 40-41]

Santosha (Contentment)

In the name of Santosha, beware of sloth, passivity, complacency, and fatalism! Rather one should plan and work for realistic goals in pursuit of common welfare, and not get perturbed by actual outcomes.

Discontentment is the result of unrealistic and selfish schemes. One should not dissipate *present* moment [gift] in favour of unrealistic hopes and expectations about future, nor in fond memories of past.[47]

In contentment, one remains committed to common well-being, without being swayed by joy and sorrow, success and failure, progress and setback, et al.

Contentment alone brings true happiness!

Not only that, one should cultivate ...

---

[46] Mental purity is the objective, but it is at best an ideal. In a later section Avidya, we shall observe that terms purity and morality are relative and evade determination.

[47] Future and past are simply figment of mind.

Tapas (Endurance)

... to stoically endure obstacles and annoyance arising in the path of yoga.

In the name of Tapas, no one is allowed to harm one's own life even. Masochist endurance is not approved – being extrinsic and pretentious.

Tapas brings about perfection of body, senses, and mind. The more inclined and prepared we are, the faster we learn life's lessons!

Svadhyaya

It means study of scriptures aimed at knowing Self. Scriptures regard Self-ignorants as doomed because they carry the enemy within them! [IU 3] They do not know themselves [Self] and therefore their objectives of self-fulfilment lead them astray![48] Therefore, one should make a resolute enquiry into Self or *Who am I?* ... Study should be faithful and critical!

Svadhyaya implants revered virtues of ideal deity, or brings in realisation of the deity as Self.

Ishvara-pranidhana (Surrender to God)

Pre-eminence of this Niyama is evident from Yoga text, *e.g.*, this Niyama *by itself* brings about perfection of Samadhi [II 45] and, in combination with Tapas and Svadhyaya, it forms 'practical path to yoga' [II 1].

---

[48] If you donot know where you are going, every road will get you nowhere. (Henry Kissinger)

No matter if it is counted as last among Yamas and Niyamas, it remains central in significance and deed. We shall revert to it in detail in section 'Surrender to God'.

Yamas and Niyamas are pivotal in self-evolution of yoga through the remaining limbs. Remember the admonition of Yoga: argument for deviation from them should be countered with sound reason. Any deviation is in fact prompted by greed, anger, and delusion with consequences of endless ignorance and pain. [II 33-4]

CHAPTER FOUR

Asana and Pranayama

❄

PHYSICO-PSYCHOLOGICAL FITNESS

Tired? Feeling hungry? Craving for food? STOP!

WE DO NOT REQUIRE AS MUCH REST AND FOOD.

Tap superior source of life energy (Pranayama) adopting a variety of physical postures (Asanas).[49] NOURISH BODY CELLS WITH OXYGEN[50] and see the miracle of yoga! ... You relax and refresh by exerting! Happiness belongs to hard working! *It is* paradoxical.

MAKE UP YOUR MIND. COUNTER EXCUSES.[51] Body is unconscious; it cannot argue and take initiative!

Breath-synchronising Asanas (*e.g.*, SUN SALUTATION) are particularly beneficial. But be regular to retain physical and emotional benefits.

BREATHE OUT DEEP [I 34] is the categorical message of Yoga. [Recall Antidote Sutras of Synopsis.]

---

49 Walking and jogging for half an hour every day in fresh air is far better than doing nothing.

50 In all serious disease states we find a low oxygen state occurring, and low oxygen in the body tissues is a sure indicator of disease. (Dr. Stephen Levine)

51 Overcome *tamas* with *sattva* and *rajas*. With **attentive physical activity**, you gain physically and also ward off inertia, depression, insanity, and ignorance (*tamas*).

Hand Positions (Mudras)

These are indeed handy positions.

Chin (Chit) Mudra Softly join tips of index finger and thumb, as shown in figure of Lotus Posture. Hands should rest on knees or thighs and palms face upward. True to its name, it stimulates intelligence.

Vayu Mudra Curl index finger and press it on the palm. It relieves pain. Vayu means wind.

Shunya Mudra Middle finger is folded on the palm and pressed. It relieves ear-related disorders. Shunya means void.

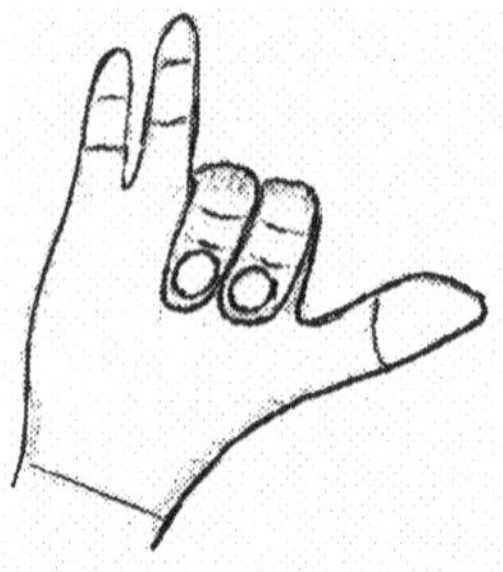

Vishnu Mudra is Vayu and Shunya Mudras together. For Pranayama, use right hand. Use little and ring fingers and thumb to pinch your own nostrils for regulating breath. [See topic Pranayama.] Thumb is used for pressing right nostril; and fingers for left. This Mudra bestows elegance and cheerfulness.

Apana Mudra Join tips of thumb and middle and ring fingers. It relieves body of impurities. It is also used while releasing offerings into sacrificial fire.

Mrita Sanjivani Mudra is Apana and Vayu Mudras together. It saves one from even life-threatening situations, like heart attack.

ঌ Asana ଓ

> *Asana* is physical posture that is steady and comfortable. It is mastered over time, with effort relaxed and mind absorbed in the Infinite or Absolute (Brahma). Asanas firm up body and eliminate annoyance of dualities of life such as hot-and-cold and pleasure-and-pain. [II 46-48]

'Steadiness' and 'comfort' attributes of Asanas are precursors of Samadhi. *Steady* posture with *steady* breathing arrests impulsivity and fickleness of mind.[52] ... Asana and Pranayama together become a plane for introspection and meditation.

Basic hints for the beginner would not be out of place. Detail is beyond the scope of this book. Serious reader should personally consult yoga teacher or refer to a good book[53] on yoga exercises.

- Ensure ventilation of your premises.
- Sleep at fixed hour and for fixed number of hours [not more than 8]. Get up well before sunrise.
- Yoga session should be soon after we get up in the morning and after routine bowel movement and oral hygiene. It can even be after bath. Early morning session ensures vitality for the whole day.
- BE RELAXED, BUT ATTENTIVE [HERE-AND-NOW]. Do not (mentally) wander off the site. Be with the moves and pauses – this stirs up higher yoga limbs!
- Carefully avoid over-enthusiasm and exercise overload. Do not be in a hurry to add exercises – wait for at least two weeks. Remember: slow and steady wins the race. Otherwise, you can exhaust yourself and quit for good!

---

[52] Agitated body and breathing are sure indicators of agitated mind.

[53] See Bibliography (Appendix E).

- Yoga session should progress from warm-up, simple postures to intense, challenging ones, and then to rest postures like Corpse Posture, then to Pranayama, and lastly to meditation. Each posture should be followed by a counter or restorative posture.
- SINCERE START, EVEN IF SMALL, WITH A FEW YOGA POSTURES — THAT IS THE KEY TO THE MIRACLE OF YOGA!

There is an amazing variety as easily to suit all age groups and people with special needs. But we discuss a few of them *viz.* Sun Salutation, Head Stand, Lotus Posture, Diamond Posture, Tree Posture, and Corpse Posture.[54] We also discuss Stationary Race.

We presume beginner fit for light exertions. During yoga session, if you experience pain or discomfort of any kind, stop, relax, and resume comfortably if you can, without any feelings of guilt and failure. It is advisable to consult physician before practising asanas.

DIAMOND POSTURE (VAJRASANA)

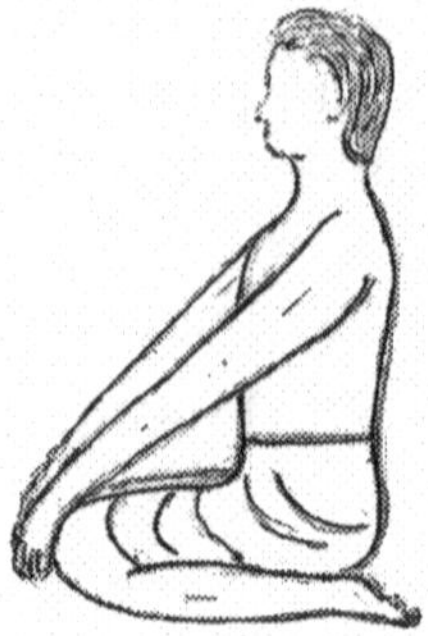

It is any-time and any-duration posture. It is beneficial after meals too. Use carpeted floor. Sit on knees with buttocks resting on heels and right toe [thumb] placed on left. Spine and head should be straight and at right angles to floor – this minimises ill effects of gravitation. Palms rest on knees. Arms are straight.

[54] Their Sanskrit names are like this: sūrya namaskāra, śīrṣa asana (or śīrṣāsana), paḍma asana (or paḍmāsana), vajra asana (or vajrāsana), ṭāda asana (or ṭādāsana), and śava asana (or śavāsana), respectively.

LOTUS POSTURE (PADMASANA)

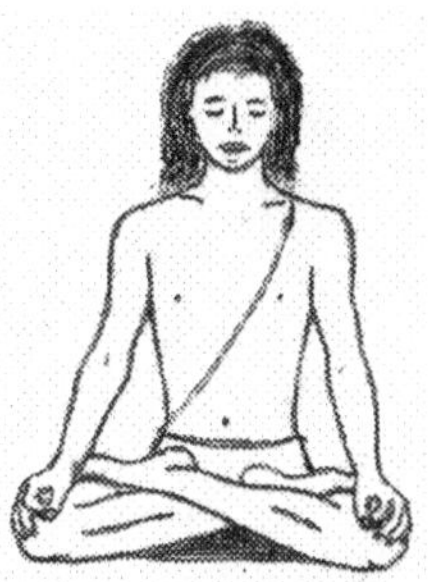

We discuss only where it differs from previous posture. Put right foot on left thigh, and left on right. Let heels be closer to navel and soles face upward, emulating the petals of a blooming lotus. Hands can be in Chin Mudra. Alternatively, place hands in the lap, palms facing up with: 1) fingers gently interlocked, or 2) one hand resting on the other. It keeps vital currents from escaping body.

SUN SALUTATION (SURYA NAMASKAR)

One round of Sun Salutation involves movement through certain simple but vital Asanas, synchronised with breathing. As Sun Salutation session of 6-11 rounds progresses, movement becomes smooth; and still postures acquire a dynamic aura. It becomes urgent to breathe faster and, in turn, to move faster between postures. It is regarded a wholesome ritual!

Beginner should not feel frustrated by early setbacks. First, try them singly; then, as a sequence.

[0] *Stand straight and Inhale.* In starting position [not shown in the figure], keep feet joined and arms dropped to sides. We stand facing east or northeast.

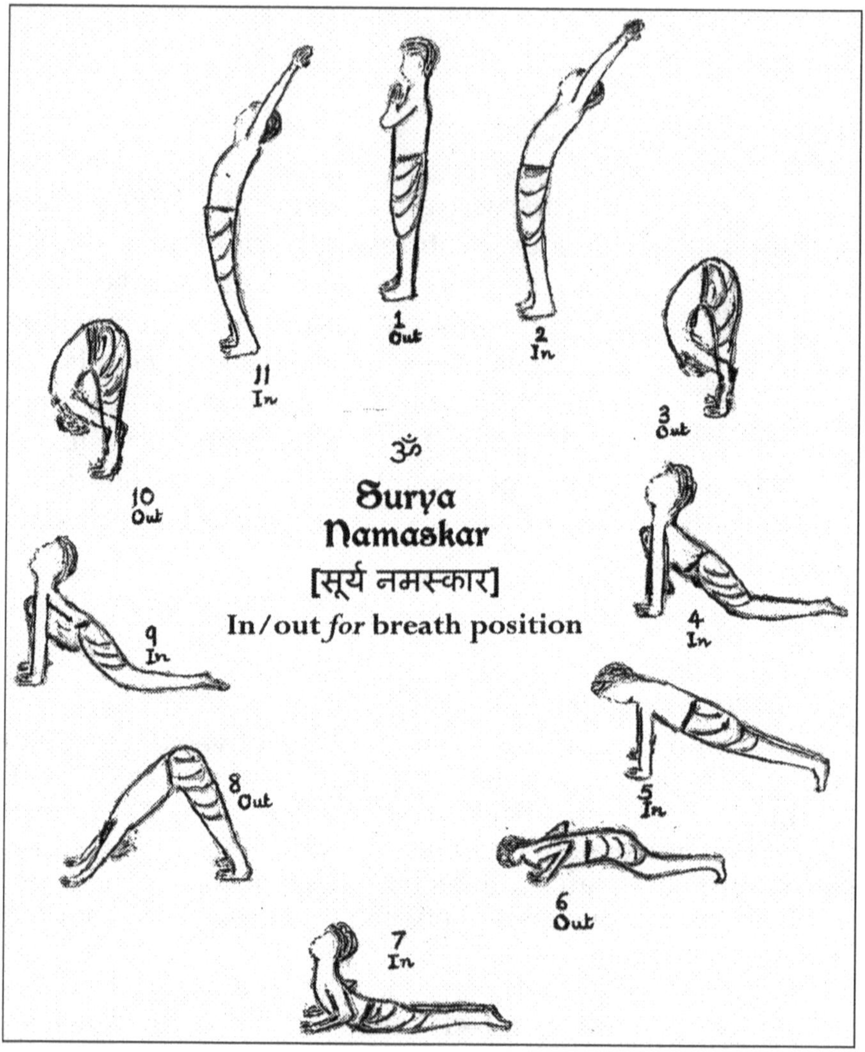

[1] *Prayer pose* Exhaling deeply, join hands in prayer pose, with forearms making a straight (horizontal) line and elbows pointing to sides.

[2] *Raised-hand prayer pose* Inhaling, raise praying hands straight up as to cover ears; and, then, along with the head, stretch back, making an arch along the back.

[3] *Fold pose* Exhaling steadily, retreat and then bend forward, ending with 1) palms resting on ground in line with the feet and 2) face as close to kneecaps or legs as practicable. Ideally, knees should not be bent. In case you need to bend knees, then try to pull hips high as far as possible while keeping palms on the ground.

[4] *Crescent pose* Inhaling and lowering body, extend right leg back as far as possible with toe pointing behind; and look up stretching your neck.

[5] *Push-up pose* Holding breath in, move left leg back along right and balance on hands and toes.

[6] *Eight-organ salute* Exhaling deeply, lower knees, chest, and forehead only, to touch the ground. Elbows point backward.

[7] *Cobra pose* Inhaling, lower whole body to the ground and start raising head, helped by push from hands. Stretch neck backward and look up. Hands support the raised upper-half of body. Elbows point backward.

[8] *Dog stretch* Exhaling thoroughly, lower your chest and then raise hips as up and backward as possible. Now start retreating steps.

[9] *Crescent pose* Inhaling, bring right foot forward between hands, stretch left leg backwards as far as possible with toe pointing behind; and look up stretching your neck. Compared to posture [4], left here is right there, and right here left there.

[10] *Fold pose* Exhaling thoroughly, bring left foot forward along right foot and resume position [3].

[11] *Raised-hand prayer pose* Inhaling, return to position [2]. Then, exhaling deeply, return to starting position [0].

In the next round, start with other, left leg in position [4].

HEAD STAND (SHIRSHASANA)

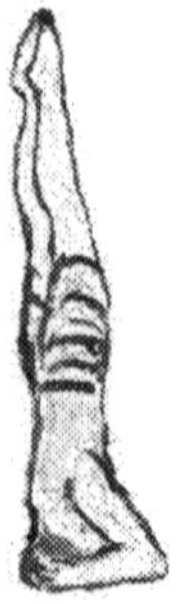

CAUTION This posture should not be attempted in conditions of high blood pressure, heart problem, pregnancy, etc. In case of doubt, consult your doctor before practising this posture. Even otherwise, it should not be attempted unless you have practised other yoga postures for at least one month and you feel you can bear the strain of inversion.

It is better to practise it initially against wall and under supervision. Start with Diamond Posture. Lock fingers and kneel forward to rest elbows on the ground, forming the shape of inverted V. Raising knees and taking body weight on toes, place front head on ground. To avoid injurious twist to your neck and spine, support head firmly from sides by finger-interlocked hands/palms. Lift legs and take body weight on firm elbows and locked palms – weight on head should be avoided or minimum. Then straighten legs above torso. Stay there for 2-3 minutes only.

It helps in defying gravity and arresting ageing. It should be followed by Tree Posture or Corpse Posture.

TREE POSTURE

Stand straight. Inhaling steadily and raising arms straight upwards to cover ears, raise yourself on toes. Hands are open and fingers point upward. Stretch your body as if you are hanging from branch of a tree. Stay there as long as you can hold breath. Then return exhaling deeply. This can be repeated several times.

CORPSE POSTURE

Lie on your back like a corpse. Close eyes and keep hands and legs straight and slightly open. Palms face upward.

Shake tense portions. Breathe attentively and relax your body. It is a restorative posture.

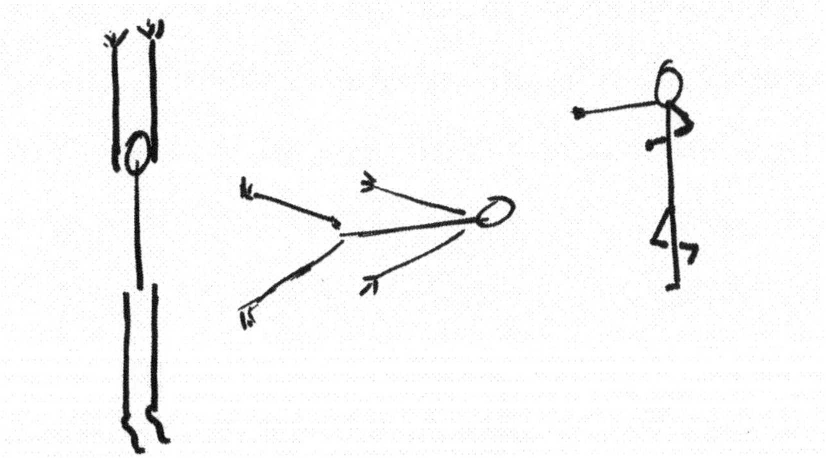

Figure Tree Posture, Corpse Posture, and Stationary Race (left to right)

STATIONARY RACE

My Yoga teacher (Ashok Kumar*ji*) recommends this one. It is simple as it involves two steps only. Its simplicity belies its advantages!

It has inbuilt Pranayama; builds cardiopulmonary efficiency; and lifts sagging spirits.

Keep thumbs enclosed in fingers throughout the race.

Step 1 Stand on left leg with left arm straight out in the style of punching someone in front. Right leg is up and right arm kept back in race action. Breath should be thrown out in this position.

Step 2 While inhaling, move to alternate position (*i.e.*, changing left with right, and vice versa).

Return to starting position with breath belched out. Let soles of feet strike buttocks if possible. Remember: breathing out should be forceful. When movement between steps gets smooth, it will mock the sight and sound of a racing steam engine!

As we progress in yoga session, there are noticed instant and assuring rewards in the form of *light* and *agile* body. There is smooth and subtle flow of breath in *both* nostrils. These are indicators of our fitness for next yoga limbs.

Pranayama

Further emerges Pranayama (life-expansive energy) from natural or arranged suspension of flow of breath. Pranayama means superior source/dimension of life energy. Along with suspension of breath is suspended mind (thinking). Benefits include: severance of identifications with objects, possessions, body, and mind; dawn of discriminative knowledge (knowledge born of Viveka); and fitness for attentiveness (higher yoga limbs). [II 49-53]

Pranayama is inbuilt in Asanas. Nevertheless, it can be practised independently and proactively.

In order to resolve mind, sit in an easy posture like Lotus Posture. Eject breath with force in 3-4 moves as in vomit (drawing stomach in); then hold it out — pressing nostrils using Vishnu Mudra (as shown in figure on the page) and pressing chin against chest. Then, when feeling urgent, release chin and fingers and recover breath in 2-3 moves. Repeat this for several times. [I 34]

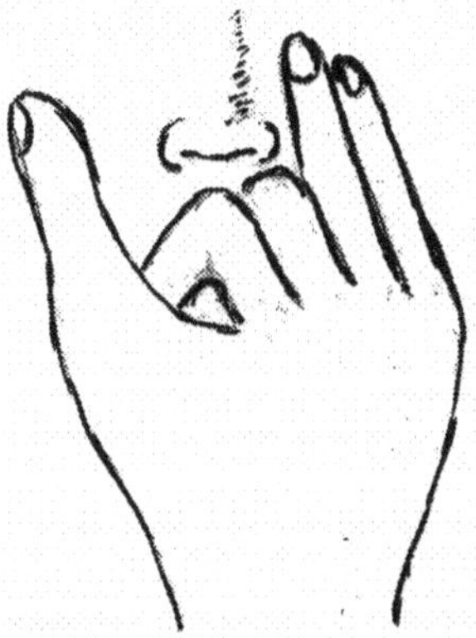

DO NOT inhale greedily, rapidly, or anxiously. It can disturb the chemistry of blood, by faster loss of carbon dioxide. You can feel dizzy! ... REMEMBER TO BREATHE OUT WELL.

You can also practise breathing out and in from one nostril at a time. Press the right nostril, then breathe out deep from left and then inhale. Then, pressing left nostril, repeat the process from right. Keep alternating. In this, we do not retain breath in or out. This is ***Anuloma Viloma Pranayama. ...***

Practising retention of breath in should come quite later. Moreover, it is optional. For retaining breath in, you should contract your perineum. The other process is similar.

Asana and Pranayama are austere and optimal way of life, conserving our resources and energies. Otherwise, we abuse resources, deprive the needy of their share, and violate the Ahimsa and Aparigraha principles. We may be eating more than what is needed! We can experience false hunger and craving for food!

Tap superior source of energy, Asana and Pranayama!

CHAPTER FOUR

Toward Samadhi

❄

OBJECTIVE AWARENESS AND FICTIVE PERSONALITY

KEY TO SAMADHI

MIND CANNOT BE ON TWO OBJECTS AT THE SAME TIME. [IV 20]

Hold mind (attention) on any physical here-now[55] object/activity of choice or on breathing. Keep returning to it. Comfortable stillness of posture facilitates it further. Breathing becomes slow, smooth, and even suspended; so does mind (thinking)! There dawn objectivity and Viveka!

> With obsession of memories [preoccupations with past and language], of inferences [assumptions and expectations], and of authorities [precedents and guides] subsided, in **Samadhi** (meditation), (1) objects meditated are seen as they are and (2) meditator is seemingly devoid of Self or his nature (*i.e.*, self-forgetful). [I 43, 48-9; III 3]

We cannot be otherwise than present [here-now]. Unfortunately, we remain mentally absent and unaware of our mental escapades!

The moment we see something, hear something, touch, taste, or smell; we turn away from it for cerebral encounter or probe and relating it to some name, meaning, purpose,

---

[55] An object far-off or not existing now can turn fanciful!

precedent, belief, dogma, antecedents, and possible issues (outcomes). In the name of rationality, the tiny, original experience gets sacrificed in flirtation. ... We stray into a maze of diversions, wicked enough to foil the thrill of an otherwise neat experience. ... This goes on every time and every moment. We go on missing life! We are unmindful of five-fold sumptuous life!

Two terms objective awareness and fictive personality define Samadhi. The two even explain each other.

Objective Awareness

It signifies many things. Objects are seen here as they are and not as they appear to us. We do not start believing at first sight! Things are seen dispassionately or as distinct from Self. Meditator is not interpreting subjectively or from selfish standpoint. He can also be called self-forgetful.

Moreover, as knowing (*seeing,* consciousness) is our nature and not the changing knowledge (*seeable*), there cannot be any obstinate and arrogant claims of knowledge.

Fictive Personality

Can one be devoid of Self or one's nature [Consciousness]? Obviously not. *Only seemingly.* Meditator here can be described as: [1] self-forgetful[56] or [2] devoid of personality. In the first case, meditator can forget his nature but cannot be devoid of it. In the second, he does not identify personality (changing face or mask; or what he thinks he is) as his true Self. ...

[Samadhi is non-judgemental witnessing (free from dogma and bias). It is being oneself.]

---

56 Having or showing no thought of self or selfish interests [Merriam Webster's Collegiate Dictionary]

Samadhi Transformation of Mind

Resuming from progress so far in previous chapters, we expect that abilities for further yoga limbs should manifest themselves by now. Devotee has acquired fitness for attentiveness. [II 53] Senses have withdrawn from their objects in **Pratyahara**, the fifth yoga limb. [II 54] Now we take up the last three yoga limbs.

In Concentration (**Dharana**), attention is held on physical, material, here-now objects/activities, instead of hypothetical or fanciful, so that one does not wander off mentally or slips into reveries! [III 1] ... Here, AWARENESS (THE THINKING SUBJECT; ATTENTION) MATTERS, NOT THE OBJECTS OF ATTENTION OR THOUGHT. Common examples of Dharana are: 1) when we see something interestedly for the first time; and 2) when we carefully read warning signs.

In Contemplation (**Dhyana**), object of attention remains uniform; at least it does not change unawares! Ideally, it is a longer, uninterrupted session of Dharana on a single object or activity. [III 2]

In the background of yoga limbs, now one notices:

- Tangible severance of identifications with thought objects;
- Thought objects getting increasingly distinguished (separate) and insignificant;
- Infrequent disturbing thoughts;
- Wider gaps between successive disturbing thoughts; and
- Growing neutrality/indifference toward thoughts and even gaps between thoughts.

One neither evades nor judges them as good or bad, but just witnesses [darshana[57]]. Dispassion brings objectivity. What were once fixations and indulgences now get objectively[58] distinguishable. Mind – that was once notoriously fickle, vacillating, and dispersed – gets ONE-POINTED (FOCUSED) AT WILL[59]. This is the beginning of Samadhi, called Samadhi transformation of mind.[60] [Revisit opening passages of the chapter.]

---

[57] *Darshana* is seeing (or knowing) and not philosophy (knowledgeable viewpoints on life; which should technically be called *drishya*).

[58] As distinct from Self or not interpreted subjectively or selfishly

[59] The qualification 'at will' is meaningful. Otherwise worry which too looks one-pointed becomes Samadhi. One does not enter or come out of worry at will. It is *not* conscious absorption.

[60] *Samadhi transformation of mind* is described in Yoga as disappearance of all-pointedness (dispersiveness) and simultaneous rise of one-pointedness, in the mind. [III 11]

Samadhi in Practice

> In a clean/ventilated place, set up a steady seat over grass, deer hide, and cotton sheet. It should be neither high nor low. [BG VI 11]

Sit in an easy, still posture like Lotus Posture or Diamond Posture and HOLD ATTENTION ON PHYSICAL OBJECT/ACTIVITY THAT APPEALS TO YOU. [Refer to Antidote Sutras of Synopsis. Objects of choice hold attention easily and reduce monotony and tedium.]

LAPSES DO NOT MATTER. There is no merit in harbouring feelings of guilt and frustration. Return to the chosen object of attention. ... Keep returning but not obsessively or with effort.

Relax obsession and effort. Step back into reflexive state and PROBE DISTRACTIONS.[61] Such probing awareness is auspicious. This abstraction works and restores composure.

Samadhi is not just focusing or concentration; it is *lila* (play)! [Recall Antidote Sutras of Synopsis.]

Alternatively, ATTEND UNMANAGED BREATH. Attune to instinctive, concomitant *So'ham* (सोऽहम्) chant[62], that resounds with every cycle of breathing – *So* with inhalation and *'ham* with exhalation. Let bygones be bygones and let forthcomings be unanticipated. Witness the *actual* breath. Be with the moment. During pauses between breaths, watch against verbalisations, opinions, and judgements. Instead,

---

[61] Consciousness is the perception of what passes in a man's own mind. (John Locke)

[62] *So'ham* means 'That I am.' Here, *So* signifies 'That Brahma or Purusha.' The chant implants in our subconsciousness the fundamental identity between individual and Universal Being (Brahma). It has been extolled as an auspicious, unchanted chant (coincident with breathing). One has just to be aware of breath moving in and out. It is natural and effortless and therefore free from any demerit or taint!

be with the moment – be here-now (mentally present). In between if necessary, just be aware of physical self and objects and passage of time. ...

There such is the *objective* awareness that objects cease to exist as they appear to us. Perceptions stop pretending as Truth. In this reflexive state, though one cannot deny Self, but still cannot objectively substantiate and describe It. Personality, property, and other preoccupations all are objectively seen as distinguished (distinct) from Self. Self is there as *knowing* and still not there in objective terms. One experiences fictive personality; ever-changing personality posing as Self is exposed! Hence the comment AS IF DEVOID OF SELF. ...

The third chapter (Vibhuti) of Yoga is an exercise in HERE-AND-NOW. This is evident from Yoga text: locational concentration (*dharana*) [III 1]; *Samyama* as dharana, dhyana, and samadhi together [III 4]; and questioning the usual notions of time[63] [III 52].

There is a story in The Mahabharata epic about Yudhishthira and his brothers, the princes in exile. They were living life of commoners. One day a beggar came to their door for alms. Yudhishthira felt pity for him and even for himself – he had nothing worthwhile to offer. He promised to help him the next day and asked him to revisit them. Beggar believed him [latter was well known for truthfulness] and went away.

Younger brother Bhima overheard all this and laughed. He picked up a drum and ran out beating it. He announced to the villagers: 'O folks, I do not believe you know someone who has conquered time. However I know. My brother Yudhishthira has conquered time. He has promised to help

---

[63] Myth of time is demolished there. Firstly, it is not correct to conceive time as collection or sequence of moments. No two moments coexist – one of the two is bound to be preceding (no more existing) or succeeding (yet to exist). In other words, one has to be non-existent. So explains Sage Vyasa. Secondly, past, present, and future are not absolute terms. Same event can be all the three for different observers.

someone tomorrow! *Time is certain for him and not contingent!'...*

After discussing essentials of Samadhi, we just make a fleeting mention of various Samadhis.

Samadhi (conscious absorption) progresses in forms of speculation, reflection, exultation (*ananda*), and self-absorption (*asmita;* I-am-ness). [I 17, 41-51 *passim.*] Speculation (or vacillation) is associated with gross objects; and reflection (or deliberation) with subtle. Each of speculation and reflection is further divided into rough and smooth. However, they are attended with potential pitfalls of Kleshas and Samskaras. As such, they are inferior.

Seedless Samadhi [*i.e.,* with Kleshas and Samskaras nipped ceaselessly] is the ultimate. ... It is synonymous with flowering of knowledge of Self. [I 16]

✵

SECTION THREE

Mind

THE MEDIUM, SEEABLE, AND CONJURER

CHAPTERS

> By virtue of its proximity to Purusha (Self) and for reasons of its existence not for itself, mind produces illusions of experience (bhoga) and fakes as Self. …
>
> [Nevertheless] one who distinguishes Self from mind and accordingly practises in life knows all beings and rules all states.[64]

Bhoga (enjoyment of objects) results from failure of Viveka; or when thoughts project themselves as truths, and objects as Self.

---

64 YS III 35, 49; IV 19

CHAPTER ONE

My Mind be of Shiva Samkalpa!

❄

In Sanskrit, shiva samkalpa means non-discriminatory good will – good will and intention for all and not just for some or even if it is majority. *Shiva* means auspicious, propitious, kind, benevolent, friendly, and agreeable. *Samkalpa* means will, fancy, and resolution – it is the way mind proceeds. Title of the chapter is a refrain of Hymn to Mind; hymn in original appears in Appendix D.

HYMN TO MIND

My mind that roams places near and far,
While awake and in dreams;
Light of lights (primary among senses), the one —
That my mind be of shiva samkalpa![65]

The faculty that executes
Courageous feats and dialectic debates;
Beginningless, the divine within beings —
That my mind ... (Refrain)

That dwells within all beings
As cognition, intelligence, 'n' drive;
The will that coaxes every act — ... (Refrain)

Genius that cognises objects
Gone-by, current, and forthcoming;
And that administers all sacrifices — ... (Refrain)

In whom all The Vedas converge
Like spokes of wheel joined to hub;
All cognitions wherein merge
and wherefrom emerge — ... (Refrain)

---

65 तन्मे मनः शिवसङ्कल्पमस्तु। (ṭan me manaḥ śivasaṃkalpamasṭu!)

> As adroit charioteer reins in horses,
> So does mind drive men;
> Sitting within and still outrunning all — … (Refrain)

Hymn is panegyric. It admires and celebrates mind as glorious, versatile, and pilot of body vehicle. … Whereas, to us, the hymn looks enigmatic! We hear of mind as wicked and profane. We can call hymn just a prayer or wish for well-being of all. …

Hymn is reproduced here to highlight an oblique but profound suggestion: the words MY MIND. Two words point to an implicit distinction between mind and Self.

Is this suggestion far-fetched? Then look at the following:

> He dwelling in mind is other than mind, whom mind does not know, for whom mind acts as body, and who controls mind from within …[66]

Here the distinction stands expressly stated.

---

[66] यो मनसि तिष्ठन्मनसोऽन्तरः, यं मनो न वेद, यस्य मनः शरीरम्, यो मनोऽन्तरो यमयति (yo manasi ṭiṣthanmanaso'nṭaraḥ, yam mano na veḍa, yasya manaḥ śarīram, yo mano'nṭaro yamayaṭi) [BU III vii 20]

Medium and Seeable

Appropriate to our level of understanding and true to the wisdom of hymn, Yoga proceeds to unravel the mystery of mind to the extent of its transcendence. [IV 15-26 *passim.*] It too distinguishes in the same way and employs two different words: **chitta** (mind) and **Chiti** (Consciousness). Chitta is the starting point – refer to definition of yoga as inhibition of chitta-processes. [I 2] However, Chiti is the end and is described as:

> Establishment in Self, where there remains no purpose of life to be fulfilled and world rolls back. [IV 34]

Mind according to Yoga plays **dual role**. Normally, it fakes/personifies as Self. Whereas in Samadhi, it is seen as distinguishable and reflecting/mirroring Self. [IV 23] Mind is knower as far as other objects are concerned – it knows (illumines) them. However, it cannot know itself and is an object of knowledge (drishya) for Self (Drashtri, Chiti, or Purusha).[67]

Now reader must have got answer for extravagant adjectives used for mind in the hymn! ... ...

Mind in Yoga is not regarded as truly reflexive! Not only it does not know itself, it also cannot be known by another mind either. Had one mind been known by another, then latter mind would require still another mind to know it. This will not end anywhere and there will be confusion of memories too. Therefore, Yoga reveals mind and mental processes as objects of knowledge of Self. [IV 18]

Hence, MIND IS NOT ME, BUT MY INTERNAL INSTRUMENT OR ACCESSORY[68] — THE CLOSEST MEDIUM. It is difficult but not impossible to distinguish it from Self!

---

[67] YS IV 18, 19, 23

[68] called अन्तःकरण (antaḥ-karaṇa)

The Conjurer

> An object is known or unknown — that depends on mind whether or not coloured by that object. [IV 17]

For me this sutra sounds exciting! Read it as: an object is known or unknown [to be existing] – that depends on mind whether or not coloured by that object. Alternatively, WHAT WE KNOW EXISTS FOR US; WHAT WE DO NOT, DOES NOT.

Isn't then knowledge a substratum for existence, and ignorance a substratum for non-existence?

In a sense, we have arrived at the fundamental philosophical equation:

EXISTENCE (SAT) = CONSCIOUSNESS (CHIT)

Yoga also explains via mind the mystery of multiplicity in life. The Rig Veda had long before spoken of unity of life, saying, 'The wise speak of one truth (existence) variously and repeatedly *viz.* Indra, Mitra, Agni, etc.' [RV I clxiv 46] However, Yoga provides cogent explanation for this paradoxical unity:

> The same object appears differently to different minds that perceive it. [IV 15]

In other words, things exist for us the way we think (perceive) and not as they really are.[69] It is fallacious to call objects perceived as real! In all fairness, they could be mental and verbal constructs or projections, or pseudo-objects.[70] THINGS PERCEIVED MAY NOT EXIST! But we believe them. Mental projections are inherently deceptive. They are personal. ... MIND IS NOT ULTIMATELY RELIABLE!

---

[69] No two people see the external world in exactly the same way. To every separate person a thing is what he thinks it is; in other words, not a thing, but a think. (Penelope Fitzgerald)

[70] I confused objects with their names; that is belief. (Jean Paul Sartre)

Constitution of Mind

Mind's constitution[71] reveals inherent conflict in its purposes:

Mind is made up of three *gunas*: namely *sattva* (illumination, knowledge), *rajas* (greed, passion, impulsion, restlessness, and becoming), and *tamas* (inertia, ignorance). Essentially, it illumines objects. However, when influenced by rajas and tamas, it loves power and possessions. When tamas dominates, it is drawn to vice, ignorance, attachment, and helplessness. When tamas subsides, it is still drawn/attracted [by excess of rajas] but now to virtue, knowledge, detachment, and power, respectively. When rajas too disappears, mind is established in its being (sattva; essence or knowledge), revealing simply Viveka[72].

---

[71] Refer to Sage Vyasa's comments on yoga sutra I 2.

[72] Viveka indeed is knowledge (non-tamas) and effortless (non-rajas)!

Be therefore careful not to rush:

- ❄ to escape or transcend mind – every effort (being rajas in nature) shall frustrate. Such escape can become a new mind game. The more intense the effort, the more you can sink into it! ... So relax effort, but remain watchful!
- ❄ to conclude that tamas (ignorance) has diminished. That could be perception! Therefore, beware or be aware!
- ❄ to claim triumph and transcendence of mind and assume an air of finality. That may be delusional and transient! Judgements change with *changing* mind![73] Drop all claims!

Understanding mind as non-self and doubting its approach as valid herald its transcendence. Yoga reaffirms this cautious approach in the following sutra:

> One who has comprehensively realised this (non-self) distinction, unreliable character, etc. of mind then ceases to cogitate or actualise Self. [IV 25]

Self is not an object of thought processes and becomings; and is rather witness of al mind games!

---

[73] All our final decisions are taken in a state of mind that is not going to last. (Marcel Proust)

CHAPTER TWO

Murky Mental Processes

❄

Yoga is inhibition (nirodha) of mental processes. [I 2]

Otherwise, the result is unnatural and unbecoming conformity (or identification). [I 3-4]

Mental processes are five: pramana (right knowledge), viparyaya (illusion), vikalpa (fancy/delusion), nidra (deep sleep), and smriti (memory). These five are further of two types: producing misery and not producing misery. [I 5-6]

Beware! Seeing is believing. Keep vigil and detachment toward mental processes. 'Unexamined life is not worth living.' (Socrates)

We are Gullible

Kids were busy scanning and admiring clear blue sky. They became curious to see an aeroplane crossing the skies. They watched its entire course except the part over bright Sun. The children were aghast – for them the aeroplane reached the Sun and still did not burn!

Unwittingly we grown-ups too harbour ignorance in beautiful, alluring forms. We are quite accustomed to error – to us it is no more abnormal or sin[74]. We do not question our mental processes.

In last chapter, we learnt mind as non-self and unreliable. Therefore it becomes imperative to be careful about its processes.

Yoga rightly admonishes us to outgrow/transcend mind and its processes. Otherwise, we can *conform* (identify with) mental processes, which eventually means: MIND WILL APPEAR AS SELF; AND THOUGHTS AND DELUSIONS APPEAR AS MEANINGFUL TRUTHS! ... In this light, our error should become obvious. Mental processes ultimately produce misery. So the sooner the mental processes are checked, the better!

This wholesale disapproval of mental processes may appear far-fetched and unappealing! Why to question every thought? ...

But there indeed lies the wisdom of Yoga. To examine it, first we need to analyse the five mental processes. [I 7-11]

---

[74] Ignorance is not innocence but sin. (Robert Browning)

∽ Examine Right Knowledge ∼

Right Knowledge, the first mental process, sounds awesome and credible. ... However, it ultimately belies our trust!

According to Yoga, right knowledge is obtained in three ways such as from direct perception, inference, and people and works of authority.

While using ***direct perception,*** we do (unknowingly) collect inaccurate or wrong information or err in judging situations. This can be due to *defective* sense-faculties, instruments, and knowledge-process. We generally tend to believe what we see (perceive). For example:

- We see Sun and Moon rising and setting and say so too. However, in reality Earth revolves around its axis and produces this illusion.
- Moon wanes and waxes but apparently.
- We may believe the stars that we see at night in the sky are there [existing now]. However, that could be wrong. Many of them must not be either existing or in the same position. ... Their information could be millions of years old. Our information here ridiculously lags behind the event!
- What happens when we partly immerse a straight stick in water? It appears bent or broken.
- Pitch of a siren appears to be changing as the siren passes by the listener.
- Rapid movement of still frames gives us the impression of motion pictures.
- Rapid movement *viz.* of sparkler produces illusory shapes.

❋ In ambiguity about the foreground and the background, image can look either a vase or two faces in profile.

❋ We see mirages over desert sands and hot roads and mistake them for water.

❋ We can see snake in the rope and bear in the bush.

❋ Moreover, it was seen in the last chapter that for us things exist to the extent and the way we know them.

Similarly, our ***inference and reasoning*** on occasions is fallacious due to unsound premises (propositions), faulty arguments, or invalid conclusions. For instance:

❋ An antecedent is not necessarily a cause of a subsequent event [*post hoc, ergo propter hoc*]. Even if it is a cause, it may not be the only cause or factor.

❋ We make hasty generalisations, based on insufficient evidence.

Authorities (acceptable sources of knowledge and information) may not be in toto relevant and valid today. We could blindly (uncritically) believe them. Most of the times, impressed by the sheer number of followers (believers) and for fear of missing it for ever, we climb on the bandwagon.

CHANGING INFORMATION AND PERSPECTIVES

What we call knowledge is no different from information[75] – that information is about something, *other*, different from observer [Self!]. This information is also particularised in space and time – it becomes irrelevant or meaningless over time or in changed situations/locations.

---

[75] Where is the wisdom we have lost in knowledge? Where is the knowledge we have lost in information? (T.S. Eliot)

We are beset with systemic and perceptual limitations. As a result our knowledge can at best be called *working hypothesis*[76]. It is bound to lose influence over time. Hypotheses are modified and even superseded. First, a thesis comes, then an antithesis, and then synthesis. At no point of time, knowledge acquired can be claimed to be perfect and conclusive. Science is in eternal pursuit of explanation for the structure and behaviour of the vast, ever-changing universe – task is daunting! … Can we then afford to be complacent and unsuspecting? [Unfortunately, we do!]

Our knowledge comprises perspectives and therefore suffers from subjectivity. These perspectives at best could be larger but not comprehensive and ultimate. … Perfect knowledge is *ideal*!

PROBLEM OF TIME LAG

All Knowledge howsoever up-to-date or latest belongs to history. For example, the stars we see may not be existing now or may have moved away from where they appear to us now. Light [information] of these stars started at least four years ago on its journey to us.[77] Even when information about event is recent, it is still historical. Much water flows down the river in the interim. … This makes us prone to error.

UNKNOWABLE SELF

No matter how ingenious we become, Self (observer) will remain unknowable (unsurpassed) – for verily in what way the Knower can be known! [BU II iv 14] … If Knower can be known, then we have to presume another Knower, for which the first Knower becomes known. This will lead to endless regress and absurdity!

---

[76] Truth in science can be defined as the working hypothesis best suited to open the way to the next better one. (Konrad Lorenz)

[77] Proxima Centauri is the nearest star, next to Sun. Its light reaches us in 4.2 years.

ONCE BITTEN, TWICE SHY

Right knowledge process is fraught with a multitude of errors. This casts a serious and reasonable doubt about validity of our knowledge. Philosopher Shankara argues:

> Rope-snake and mirage-water do not exist except in our knowledge or mind. ... So too experiences waking or dream are virtual! [Appendix B]

We shall discuss this later in chapter 6.2.

It is absurd to believe as ultimate what one sees (knows).

SEEING IS NOT BELIEVING.

Other Mental Processes

Illusion, the second mental process, is a false impression of actual object (stimulus). Whereas **fancy**, third mental process, is purely a verbal or mental construct. In fancy, objects are not there; an aura around pseudo-objects is created. Fantasies, delusions, hallucinations, phobias, dreams, and even daydreams are fancies by nature.

Memory is the fourth mental process. Memory, by nature, centres on past experience ... So how far it can fit with the present or actuality! To be in memories is like living physically in the present but mentally in the past.

Memories are said to settle over time into fixed, definite tendencies (samskaras). They thus feed vicious Klesha-Karma-Phala-Samskara cycle (in short, Klesha- chain or cycle). ...

Memories prejudice and trap the unwary. Therefore, relax obsession with memories. Clutter of memories can hold one back from Samadhi. [I 43]

Irony with us is that we keep believing our mental processes as valid and authentic. Whereas most of the times those turn out to be our fantasies, illusions, delusions, superstitions, irrational beliefs, and what not. WE FAIL IN RIGHTLY RECOGNISING/DISTINGUISHING MENTAL PROCESSES! We are duped by our own mental processes. We need to be wary and discerning!

Now we come to the fifth mental process, **sleep**. It is dreamless or non-REM[78] sleep. Compared to other mental processes, it is innocent, undisruptive, and relaxing. Sleep according to Yoga is based on the 'notion of non-existence' [I 10] or on the thought of no other (or thought of

[78] Rapid-eye-movement

no thought). In sleep, 'other' of waking and dream states disappears *mentally*.

Doesn't sleep simulate Samadhi? For reasons of absence of duality and sorrow! In line with holy assurance: neither sorrow nor delusion can smite the wise that sees oneness everywhere! [IU 7]

It may simulate. It is Samadhi by default! ...

Yoga is categorical in calling sleep a mental process. Unlike Samadhi, sleep is notional and casual (random). It appears and disappears on its own (unconsciously). Moreover, it lacks conviction of oneness. Hence, it is not Samadhi. ...

In Kaivalya or Samadhi, conviction of oneness (or no-other) abides – there all dualities are seen as reflections in the lake of mind! ...

'What I Know' is Ultimately False!

In the last chapter, mind was seen as playing dual role – it is 'knower' for other objects and an object (knowable) for Self (Drashtri). Further, it was described as changeable, vacillating, and fickle. This changeability and role-playing of mind makes it unreliable. Therefore, there is merit in constant vigilance against mental processes.

In the dual role, knowledge of mind as knower about other objects remains SUBJECTIVE. Whereas mind itself being an object of Self is incompetent to reflect Self. Or mind is ignorant about Self. ... Either way, its knowledge remains questionable. Hence when I believe, 'I know something,' *I know* part of belief remains ever valid[79] but *something* turns out to be illusory, deceptive, and elusive. What I know is ultimately false![80] For example, beauty, morality, pleasure, reality, et al remain elusive in universal and objective terms!

Yoga is unrelenting. It ridicules belief in anything as true or right! Reader has to wait until a later section Avidya. Better, beware until then and not to yield to believing whatever seen and experienced!

Surprisingly, this paradoxical postulate gets support in such affirmations, as 'I know nothing except the fact of my ignorance.' (Socrates)

---

[79] Consciousness is my inalienable nature.

[80] Ignorance can be called *my* or *personal* knowledge. No wonder, ignorance thrives in the guise of knowledge. ... If we sincerely and unpretentiously admit our ignorance, we can be delivered!

SECTION FOUR

Surrender to God

ISHVARA-PRANIDHANA

IN QUEST OF IDENTITY AND UNITY

From surrender to God comes perfection of Samadhi (or yoga). [II 45]

CHAPTERS

CHAPTER ONE

Or from Surrender to God (Lord)

❄

Title of the chapter does look unusual. However, those familiar with Yoga text will immediately recognise it and appreciate its appropriateness. It is in fact a Yoga Sutra (23rd of Quarter I *Samadhi*).

Prayer (with surrender within) is customarily regarded as meritorious. The title should serve as a gentle reminder in Yoga style and leave an enduring impression in the mind of reader to drop before God, or rather drop bounds of ego and realise *Whole* (*Brahma*) within!

All of us proudly profess ourselves as theists but overlook obligations of theism. ... If God is, then how can we be separate from Him? How can we justify divisions and treat others unfairly? How can we think of harming life? How can we betray and cheat others? How can we be greedy and wasteful? How can we fight in the name of religion? ... All this is repugnant to theism.

If God is, then all beings are His manifestation; nothing else exists. ALL IS DIVINE. And yoga becomes actuality instantly, without any effort! However, that is not the case with us.

Yoga prepares and persuades devotees into surrender to and trust in God. Surrender ultimately brings about:

- realisation of noumenon self and removal of obstacles in the path of yoga [I 29];

- perfection of Samadhi (or yoga) [II 45], and
- [combined with Tapas and Svadhyaya] weakening of Kleshas (Miseries). [II 1-2]

'Surrender to God' is favourite of Yoga.[81] The word 'or' in the title simply indicates that this yoga approach is optional – one among alternatives mentioned in Yoga for realising and perfecting Samadhi (yoga). Yoga can be realised otherwise, independently too. ...

WHY SURRENDER!

- Surrender (*give in*) is natural, real; whereas choice, possession, and doership (kartritva) are hypothetical.
- We need to outgrow individuality and personality; and
- We need to realise Lord [God] as self.
- These will be taken up in the next chapters.
- *No-Lord* philosophy leads to self-doubt, fatalism, and anarchy.

---

[81] YS I 23-29 and YS II 1-2, 32, 45

CHAPTER TWO

In Surrender to Him, Enjoy!

❄

INVOLUNTARY LIFE

All this is for habitation by the Lord (*i.e.*, Isha-vasya), whatsoever is individual universe of movement in the universal motion. By that renounced thou shouldst enjoy[82]; lust not after any man's possession.

Doing verily works in this world (and not refraining from them) one should wish to live a hundred years. Thus it is in thee and not otherwise than this; action cleaves not to a man.

Above renderings are by Sri Aurobindo. Original hymns appear in Appendix D.

Lord seated within, O Arjuna, moves all men like machines;
However, men get deluded and deem – it is *they* who move.[83]

As a principle, possessions, choice, and authority rest in *Lord* – whosoever He be! That enquiry can go on, but let surrender happen first. In true surrender, one partakes (enjoys) the authority and glory of Lord.

---

[82] Or in surrender to Him, enjoy (ţena ţyakţena bhuñjīţhāḥ). *Enjoy* is in command sense.

[83] ईश्वरः सर्वभूतानां हृद्देशेऽर्जुन तिष्ठति।
भ्रामयन् सर्वभूतानि यन्त्रारूढानि मायया॥
īśvaraḥ sarvabhūţānām hṛḍḍeśe'rjuna ţiṣthaţi;
bhrāmayan sarvabhūţāni yanţrārūdhāni māyayā. [BG XVIII 61]

Concept *Lord* and Implications

The hymn admonishes us to see all this changing world, in principle, as pervaded by Lord.

Whether we accept God (Lord) as reality or concept, result invariably is the same. Either way, we are His servants and instruments and accordingly true and obedient to His commands. ... Servants do not have choice and do not oblige by doing – they in fact are under obligation to do. ... When choice is not there, understandably there cannot be any blame! ... In surrender, choice, karma (actions), doership (kartritva), and fruits – all collapse.[84]

What about possessions! Do not covet anybody's possessions. ... After all, those possessions are whose property![85] Nobody's – Lord is the ultimate possessor. ... We cannot therefore boast of or be greedy of possessions. We could at the most be trustees or custodians!

Otherwise than this just does not hold. Recite the hymns and remember that possession, choice, and authority vest in the Lord. Let thus surrender happen. In true surrender, one partakes (enjoys) the authority and glory of Lord!

In surrender, we do and still we do not. We do but are not defiled by good and bad deeds. [Alternatively, we seemingly do!] In surrender lie true liberation and enjoyment!

Unfortunately, illusion (Maya) is the lot of others who believe and behave otherwise. ... Because they go against nature – surrender is natural, agreeable, and unarranged.

---

[84] *Cf.* BG V 14.

[85] This is the undertone of the phrase *kasyasviḍḍhana* of the opening hymn.

Involuntary Life

If we examine our life carefully, we will be shocked to find that there is no ultimate/genuine choice and volition in life. From beginning to end, our every choice – if we are bent upon calling it a choice – is subject to many conditions and restrictions. Suppose we are given a certain sum to spend in our own way. Then, the definite sum at our disposal; our acquired tastes; the information available about products and services that can be purchased; ideological compulsions; and so on – such a horde of restrictions makes choice a sham! [86]

Moreover, if choices are given to us, they cannot be called choices!

We believe and boast of choice. This is a fallacy – in reality, we rarely act on our own. We compulsively react or respond to external stimuli.[87] ... No matter how we justify our responses – instinctual or emotional, destined or rational, good or bad – COMPULSION REMAINS CENTRAL TO OUR EVERY MOTIVATION. If malice, rancour, and wantonness are compulsions of some people, then compassion and self-discipline of others.

The Bhagavad Gita explains our every action as UNAVOIDABLE OR ALLOTTED.[88] We remain under obligation in doing and in non-doing as well.[89] However, in ignorance, we exercise choice and act and are defiled too by good and bad deeds!

---

[86] ... decisive choice is seldom the latest choice in the series. More often than not, it will turn out to be some choice made relatively far back in the past. (A. J. Toynbee)

[87] Even internal stimuli are external.

[88] kārya karma (कार्य कर्म)

[89] All are helplessly driven to action. (*kāryaṭe hi-avaśaḥ karma sarvaḥ*) [BG III 5]

Ex ante or ex post – choices are notional, hypothetical! Just recognise this compulsion of life – this will transform and liberate!

Yoga affirms this. According to Yoga, excess of natural factors is responsible for producing transformations into another life-state or form. [IV 2] ... Seer Self neither produces nor undergoes transformations. He supervises and is not an agent of works. THINGS HAPPEN NOT BECAUSE OF US BUT IN SPITE OF US!

> Once a king was on a tour of his state and had gone far away from the capital. On a lonely path, he saw a hoary man carrying on his head a relatively big load. It was difficult for old man to walk. King was moved by his plight. He asked his charioteer to stop. He offered the old man ride to his place. The old man was shy of this botheration to the king. However, when insisted further, he timidly sat in the chariot. To king's amazement, the old man would not take load off his head! Old man submitted that it was enough that royal chariot carried him; he would not put additional burden on the chariot of His Majesty![90] ...

So too we ignorantly believe we do. We mistakenly assume choice, ownership, authority, and agency. We forget we are mere players.[91]

In involuntariness of life, surrender and enjoyment become reality.

---

[90] This humorous story was narrated by Osho in his discourse on The Isha Upanishad.

[91] All the world's a stage,
And all the men and women merely players:
They have their exits and entrances;
And one man in his time plays many parts,
His acts being seven ages. (William Shakespeare)

CHAPTER THREE

Prayer

❄

CONFESSION AND CALL

O Savitri (Sun, Creator), eject all vices from us; replace them with what is auspicious (good)! [1]

All should be happy and rid of adversities!
Let auspicious vistas open to all; ill luck nonesoever's lot! [2]

O Prajapati (Lord of Creatures), none other than Thou
Embodies all these bountiful creations (forms[92]);
Desires with which we pray Thee, we all [not I alone] may earn those!
We be lords [and not covetous or slaves] of riches! [3]

Lead me from unreal to real;
Lead me from darkness (ignorance) to light (knowledge);
Lead me from death to immortality! [4]

---

[92] Word *rūpa* (form, manifestation) appears in The Yajur Veda, instead of word *jāṭa* (born or creation) that is used in The Rig Veda. This perhaps was intended to suggest the illusory character of world.

The foregoing and other prayers at the end of chapter are given in original in Appendix D.

Divinity is invoked in prayer [1] for bestowing on us 'what is auspicious (good)' and not what we believe as auspicious. Prayer seeks His will or wish and not personal. This is true surrender.

In prayer [2], welfare is prayed for *all*; ill fare for *none*! The word 'all' (*sarva*) is significant.

Monotheism is central; different gods as in prayers [1] and [3] represent different aspects of the same divinity.

The prayer [4] would be discussed in the chapter.

☙ Individual, Prayer, and Surrender ❧

We can believe in God, but do not accept everything as Divine and practise accordingly. For us, multiplicity of life is real. It is perhaps premature to appreciate life as one and real-like! … There lies our need for prayer and confession. Prayer is a call for yond.

Only prayer distinguishes man from animals. It reminds him of his insignificance[93] and engenders in him humbleness, which can lift him to the height of divinity. … Prayer has ever sustained humanity.

We carry wrong notions about prayer and accordingly pray seasonally or occasionally (*e.g.*, in times of need and distress, or when we feel vanquished in the battle of life). We pray for favours from Heaven. [Per chance, this method may have succeeded!] Our prayer is sad, selfish, and plaintive. Lastly, prayer is addressed to someone outside or separate.

Real prayer is an expression of deep understanding of life and works as self-reminder. We should pray because we as individuals have physical and intellectual limitations and failings. AN INDIVIDUAL IS OF COURSE DISINCLINED TO OUTGROW HIS INDIVIDUALITY. …

Prayer ideally brings about *enlightened* surrender. Alternatively, to pray is to recognise reality and potency of the Yoga means *Surrender to God*. Prayer inspires man to realise Universal Being within him. Otherwise, he as individual is tempted to accept *his* approach and perspective as the only right and comprehensive!

---

93 The significance of man is that he is insignificant and is aware of it. (Carl Becker)

Lead me from Falsehood to Truth!

Upanishadic prayer [4] is particularly taken up because, besides its inspirational appeal, it embodies unity and enlightened surrender. Without enlightened surrender, whole remains unrealised and ego[94] [part of world] remains in turmoil[95] with world.

The prayer signifies that unless we diagnose our disease and develop insight into it, treatment is not possible. Otherwise, we live in fool's paradise deluged by unreal, darkness (ignorance), and death (uncertainty and change). Life will eventually be full of falsehood, suffering, and frustration! ...

Prayer infuses optimism; it inspires us of our need and potential to transcend duality and death. ... It prays for knowledge; for one knowingly cannot err![96] The prayer admonishes us to IDENTIFY (RECOGNISE) UNREAL, DARK (IGNORANCE), AND MORTAL WITHIN US IN ORDER TO TRANSCEND THESE. [This much, to my mind, is sufficient and a good beginning!]

In our ignorance, we go on nursing sweet delusions. One such delusion is that scriptures are meant for others and we need not follow them. How can we accept that we are ignorant and need knowledge for our sake? ...

Scriptures are meant for us only – who remain greedy, even about spiritual possessions! Scriptures go on reminding us, in different ways and in newer versions, but we go on ignoring. Only wise and enlightened truly

---

[94] Ego is an idea of Self comprising mostly non-self (*drishya*). Our salvation lies in peeling the coverings of ego. These coverings are mistaken for real Self.

[95] This turmoil stems from ignorance and therefore can not last for ever. Rather it does not exist!

[96] All wrong-doing is involuntary [unknowingly]. (Socrates)

appreciate the value of scriptures. However, for ignorant the bell in church signals death of others only![97]

The scriptures want us to know ourselves or our Self because, unfortunately, in our notion of Self much is non-self and mortal! Prayer gently admonishes us to shed this non-self.

---

[97] Never send to know for whom the bell tolls; it tolls for thee. (John Donne)

From Duality to Reality

Are dualities of life dual? This predicament of duality is no different from the one here:

> Once a professor of philosophy confessed to his students that half of what he taught them was dubious. The students were perplexed.[98] The professor further added to their dismay. He could not specify the particular dubious half!

We who do not know what false is do not know truth. ... This is applicable to all our everyday experiences *viz.* light and darkness, pleasure and pain, good and bad, and so on. For instance, we can feel fed up in excess of pleasure, because we forget pain and lack perspective. ... WE KNOW EITHER BOTH OR NEITHER.

The prayer makes it imperative on us to understand duality and unity together!

If we scrutinise dualities like pleasure and pain, good and bad, beauty and ugliness, knowledge and ignorance, et al we find them notional and relative.

Each duality forms a continuum comprising arbitrary, indeterminate points. For example, let us look at **pleasure-pain continuum** in the form of line shown below, extending both sides without end. Every point on line represents a life possibility giving pleasure or pain. As such, possibilities are endless, so is the number of points on line. This line is ordered in the sense that any life possibility to the right of another is relatively (in comparison) pleasurable. For example, B is more pleasurable than A.

---

98 The statement 'I am lying' is true if and only if it is false. (Bertrand Russell)

This scheme is an over-simplification of life but insightful. It exposes limitations of duality and comparative approach. It leaves life possibilities as ambiguous and vague. No point on line can be termed pleasure or pain in definite terms, because this depends on our reference point on the line. Let us elucidate it. A and B both can be called pleasure with reference to any point like P to the left of both A and B. Similarly, A and B both can be called pain with reference to a point Q to the right of both A and B. Still, when we consider (compare) the points A and B with each other, we call the more pleasing/preferred B as pleasure and less pleasing/preferred A as pain. ... Thus, pleasure and pain do not remain individually distinguishable – PLEASURE AND PAIN ARE NOT ABSOLUTE EXPERIENCES.[99] Pleasure exists in contrast to pain (its opposite experience). By itself, pleasure is not pleasure, and pain is not pain. HOWEVER, WE CREATE DUALITY, MAKE COMPARISONS, AND DERIVE WICKED PLEASURE.[100]

Pain P A B Q Pleasure

A primary student could be intelligent in comparison to his classmates, but still ignorant in comparison to a graduate. By himself, neither is intelligent or ignorant.

Similarly, whenever a lie exists, it does not exist independent of truth. A pure lie cannot be believed; it is neither reasonable nor probable and fails at its very birth. Can we believe a hair with horns? It is fanciful!

Likewise, change in life is recognised in relation to something slow-changing or not-changing, and not by itself. Writings in chalk (white) are visible only on the black board. A contrasting backdrop is needed for any cognition! ...

---

[99] Two ends which are not in sight (or not *seeable*) can be theoretically called absolute experiences.

[100] We are so made, that we can only derive intense enjoyment from a contrast, and only very little from a state of things. (Sigmund Freud)

On careful scrutiny, dualities cannot persist in the usual sense any longer. Duality of the prayer too is apparent and at best a starting point! It is meant to be transcended!

The duality of prayer suggests that we cannot know Truth without completely understanding false[101]. In case we admit degrees or gradations in knowledge of truth, then truth is known only to the extent falsehood is exposed. ... Hence, when we know unreal, death, and ignorance in their entirety, then so are revealed their opposites to us. APPREHENSION OF IGNORANCE ALONE BECOMES TRANSCENDENCE OF IGNORANCE (i.e., enlightenment). In knowledge of our ignorance (Avidya) lies our Liberation (yoga). We shall take up this in section Avidya.

O God, lead me from ignorance to enlightenment and help me in identifying and grasping ignorance (Avidya)! I am helpless even in unmasking my ignorance; my views are *my* views – limited, partial, perspectives. I am tempted to name them as vision or truth.[102] Lead me from ignorance to enlightenment lest ignorance should blind and mislead me anymore! ...

---

[101] Logically, truth of a proposition and falsity of its negation are equivalent.

[102] Man tends to treat all his opinions as principles. (Herbert Agar)

MORE PRAYERS ...

We meditate on glorious Lord Savitri.
He may stimulate our intelligence! [1]

O gods, we may hear only what is auspicious!
O performers of sacrifice [yajña],
We may see only what is auspicious!
As long we live, we may have sturdy bodies
And promote well-being of all! [2]

One God in all manifestations —
We may see Him in all for hundred years;
We may live up to His will for hundred years;
We may hear Him for hundred years;
We may preach about Him for hundred years;
We may not be hapless for hundred years;
This may continue even beyond! [3]

Salutation to Personification of Composure and Bounty!
Salutation to Bestower of Composure and Bounty!
Salutation to Auspicious and Benevolent *par excellence*! [4]

O Three-eyed Lord (Tryambaka), we pray
For triumph over Great Death;
So we be delivered from mortal
But we may never separate from the immortal;
Like musk melon on leaving stem retains the nectar. [5]

O god Agni, knowing all things that are manifested, lead us by the good path to the felicity; remove from us the devious attraction of sin. To thee completest speech of submission we would dispose. [6] [Translation of last hymn is by Sri Aurobindo.]

Lead me from falsehood to truth!

CHAPTER FOUR

God and My Identity

❄

Lord **is described as:**

That has gone abroad [in all] — That which is bright, bodi-less, without scar of imperfection, without sinews, pure, unpierced by evil. The Seer (*kavi*), the Thinker, the One who becomes everywhere (Realiser), the Self-existent has ordered objects perfectly according to their nature from years sempiternal. [Sri Aurobindo's rendering of The Isha Upanishad hymn]

[Each object holds in itself law of its being (Lord). Adjectives Seer and Thinker are His unmistakable signs.]

Special/supreme [universal] **Purusha** [Being within all beings] untouched by the chain of Kleshas (Miseries), Karmas (works), Phalas (fruits), and Samskaras (impressions);

In whom lies ultimate intelligence;

Guru (mentor) within, uninterrupted in time, and having guided even the most ancient tradition of teachers; and

Worthy of invoking and intoning as syllabic sound *Om* (ॐ) <u>and</u> worthy of realising as Self and witness of (and distinct from) three states/roles: waking, dream[103], and sleep[104]. [Yoga sutras I 24-29]

Then, changeless noumenon Self (Consciousness, Purusha) is grasped and obstacles in the path of yoga wither.

---

103 Including daydreams, delusions, and hallucinations

104 Non-Rapid Eye Movement phase of sleep

☙ Purusha: Individual and Universal Being ❧

Every individual remains in search of true identity in order to align life to an enduring purpose. In Yoga terminology, the ultimate objective of life is stated as Purusha-khyati (knowledge of Self).

Yoga satisfies this quest of the devotee through the principle of God (Ishvara) and by revealing in him His reflection. According to Yoga, GOD IS PURUSHA ONLY; QUALIFICATIONS ARE PREDICATES OF PURUSHA.[105] Let us elaborate it, by drawing upon evidence from other authorities as well.

- *Purusha* stands for consciousness, intelligence, and being within all beings. It is stated to be this entire universe [all that yet hath been and all that is to be][106] and is therefore individuals too. Yoga uses the term in both senses. Knowledge of this Purusha alone is adored as leading to transcendence of death. [YV xxxi 2, 18]
- *Knowing* is within us all – this is the irrefutable evidence of His pervasiveness and participation. 'No other knower than Him is there! … He is your Self, the inner controller, the immortal. Everything else than Him is mortal.'[107] …
- Instead of special/supreme, adjective *universal* of Lord is preferable. The adjective in original sutra

---

105 If individual is seen to be touched (or affected) by Miseries and so on, this is the result of belief (out of ignorance) in the truth of Miseries and so on. Or if individual sees himself as subordinate (and not supreme), he has forgotten his true identity.

106 पुरुष एवेदँ सर्वं यद्भूतं यच्च भव्यम् (puruṣa eveḍaṃ sarvam yaḍbhūṭam yachcha bhavyam.) [YV xxxi 2]

107 नान्योऽतोऽस्ति द्रष्टा / विज्ञाता … एष त आत्मान्तर्याम्यमृतः। अतोऽन्यदार्तम्। (nānyo'ṭo'sṭi ḍraṣṭā/vijñāṭā … eṣa ṭa āṭmānṭaryāmyamṛṭaḥ. aṭo'nyaḍ ārṭam.) [BU III vii 23]

means 'excluding nothing.' [Adjective special/supreme gives impression of categories of Purusha!]

- ❄ God is the eternal and universal guide (*guru*) and leader [*Agni*] within us all.
- ❄ According to The Mandukya Upanishad, OM SIGNIFIES ATMAN [INDIVIDUAL SELF] that: (1) traverses three states of waking, dream, and sleep [which project various objects and experiences (bhogas) for Him] and (2) is still unaffected, untouched, and taintless. The Upanishad reveals mystic relationship between the three states and the three constituent letters *a, u,* and *m* of Om. ... Thus, concept of Lord (Ishvara) and chant (japa) of Om work to reveal true identity and provide perspective of life. These implant in us true Drashtri (Self), distinct from Drishya.

In Yoga, God is not hypothetical or ideal, but realisable as actual (undeniable) Self! Knowing or consciousness is His unmistakable signature. That is what the word Purusha signifies!

Same or Similar! One or Onelike!

A doubt can linger! Is individual Self same as (one with) God? Or similar to God? One or onelike! ...

It is premature for the reader to assert or deny either! To assert first is more authoritative and definitive! ...

Scholars and scriptures have shown predilection for the first (unity).[108] All distinctions are analytical [perceptional] in nature! The Rig Veda proclaims:

> One existence is oft spoken of by seers in a variety of ways.[109]

The Gita lauds fair-minded people as wise — who do not favour and victimise anyone, whether it is learned and becoming Brahmin, cow, elephant, dog, or untouchable![110] ...

---

108 *eka-tva* (one/unity), *avibhāga/avibhakta* (undivided) [BS IV iv 4; BG XVIII 20]

109 एकं सद्विप्रा बहुधा वदन्ति। (ekaṃ saḍ viprā bahuḍhā vaḍanṭi.) [RV I clxiv 46]

110 पण्डिताः समदर्शिनः। (paṇḍiṭāḥ samaḍarśinaḥ.) [BG V 18]

Apart from that, Atman (Self) has been quite often used as alternative expression for Universal Being:

> The Purusha there, That I am.[111] [IU 16]
>
> Verily, in the beginning all this was Self, one only.[112]
>
> That is Real (satya). He is the Self (Atman). That thou art.[113]
>
> To wise for whom Self (Atman) alone has become all beings;
> To such seer of unity, what delusion or what sorrow clings![114]

Yoga endorses this by using such terms as KAIVALYA **(meaning 'aloneness' or absolute unity). ... Divisions, differences, and multiplicity are virtual!**

✵

---

111 योऽसावसौ पुरुषः सोऽहमस्मि। (yo'sāvasāu puruṣaḥ so'ham asmi.)

112 आत्मा वा इदमेकमेवाग्र आसीत्। (āṭmā vā iḍam ekamevāgra āsīṭ.) [AU I 1] This translation is by F. Max Müller.

113 तत्सत्यं, स आत्मा, तत्त्वमसि। (ṭaṭ saṭyam, sa āṭmā, ṭaṭṭvamasi.) [CU VI viii 7]

114 यस्मिन्सर्वाणि भूतान्यात्मैवाभूद्विजानतः। तत्र को मोहः कः शोक एकत्वमनुपश्यतः॥
(yasmin sarvāṇi bhūṭānyāṭmāivābhūḍ vijānaṭaḥ; ṭaṭra ko mohaḥ kaḥ śoka ekaṭvam anupaśyaṭaḥ.) [IU 7]

SECTION FIVE

Avidya

Ignorance of Reality

WATCH AGAINST PARADOXES!

CHAPTERS

CHAPTER ONE

Knowledge and Ignorance

❄

We are keen for higher/liberating knowledge (Vidya) but unfortunately remain trapped in the opposite. This is so because we do not know Avidya and Vidya together.[115] All our life we try to learn things to do – but that does not deliver us from trouble.[116] However, if we can know WHAT NOT TO DO – or if we know Avidya – we reap dual benefits: knowledge becomes complete and we are saved from great trouble. Without completely knowing 'what not to do' we remain prone to error!

AVIDYA WHEN IGNORED IS KLESHA (MISERY), and on its apprehension we escape pain and death.

Some may argue that ignorance is bliss. That is not correct. Ignorance clouds or holds back right knowledge and information; and creates an illusion of knowledge. An unpleasant illusion is an instant punishment. Whereas a pleasant one turns into misery when busted. Either way, illusion is evil!

In ignorance, we may be deluded to take recourse to intoxication and drugs (*i.e.*, tamas) and feel relieved of everyday woes and worries. However, this works only as long as influence of the drugs lasts. With time and

---

115 *Cf.* IU 14.

116 In addition, *doing* creates a conceited sense of agency (kartritva, doership) and grandiose – that obscures true understanding of Self.

habituation, influence fades. [After all, consciousness is our nature!] ... Intoxication does not solve problems, but only defers them for a while. In the interim, problems could remain unresolved and multiply. We try to avoid problems – that is cowardice! Regular avoidance worsens the problem. Ignoring does not help us, because according to Yoga ignorance is cause of misery and pain.

It is critical to understand Avidya comprehensively!

CHAPTER TWO

Root Klesha (Misery)

❄

> Klesha [rather Avidya] lies at the root of our merit-demerit residuum/reservoir.
>
> As long as root is there, fruits are inevitable. Accordingly, we experience births, life spans, and pleasure-pain seesaw. [II 12-13]

In Yoga Klesha (Misery) is the technical name given to intellectual, emotional, and instinctive weaknesses to which human beings remain prone. **Kleshas are five**, namely: *Avidya* (Ignorance of Reality), Egoism (*asmita*), Attachment (*raga*), Hatred/Aversion (*dvesha*), and Yearning for Life (*abhinivesha*). These are called Miseries because they bring misery with them. [YS II 2-15 *passim*.]

Yoga undertakes to help in realisation of Samadhi and simultaneous attenuation of above Kleshas. [II 2]

Even among these five, AVIDYA IS REGARDED THE ROOT MISERY, being breeding ground for the latter (four) in all their forms – whether dormant, weakened, intercepted in time, or active (current). In other words, last four Miseries stem from Avidya as its special cases. ... Then the question can arise why they are enumerated alongside Avidya. Perhaps Avidya lurks, survives elimination attempts, and is too formidable to be grasped and addressed singly. ...

Avidya, the primary Misery, can be described as Ignorance of Reality. Precisely, it is PERCEPTION OF PERMANENCE, PURITY, PLEASURE, AND SELF IN WHAT INDEED IS NOT. It is a deep-seated misconception. [We revert to it in detail in the next two chapters.]

Egoism, the second Misery, stands for erroneous and illusive identity – somewhat oneness with mind and its processes [*i.e.*, with non-self]. It is a mistaken notion of self.

Here, by virtue of their proximity, cognition faculties (sense organs, mind, and intellect) and their objects (thoughts) are mistakenly identified as Self. This identification is analogous to REFLECTIONS ON WATER – water [if it too had an ego or were to lose perspective] will mistake itself as the objects reflected in it, sometimes as Sun, sometimes as Moon, sometimes clouds, sometimes passers-by, sometimes as nothing, and sometimes confused [on getting agitated by winds]. ... Water has forgotten its nature of *reflection*.

In egoism, we too lose perspective and forget our nature *consciousness*. We become reflective, moved, and agitated like water. Media distort the message and are regarded as Self.

Egoism manifests in statements like:

I AM SOMEBODY WHO POSSESSES OR CAN DO SUCH AND SUCH THINGS ...
I ALONE AM RIGHT OR KNOW.

Claim of humbleness too is egoistic! Self-portraits are coloured and misleading.

Egoism is ignorance *unless consciously checked.*

However, here identity with instrumental faculties alone is seen as erroneous and miserable. What about identity with objects? That too is identification with non-self! ... Explanation for excluding it is that to us things are not things as they are, but as we see them. As such, identity with objects is identity with thought-objects. ... For instance, when one says one possesses houses, cattle, and wealth, one is simply nursing egoistic notions of person and property.[117]

Attachment, the third Misery, is ignorance too, because attachment stems from pleasure. What one likes, one would be drawn to it and can be greedy about it.

However, PLEASURE IS A PARADOX OF LIFE[118] [chapter 5.4]. ... Therefore, there is not much hope in attachment; it brings in pain only.

Aversion/Hatred, the fourth Misery, is also ignorance. Recourse to aversive avoidance of pain too is frustrating and painful! The argument is the same as for pleasure or attachment.

Yearning for Life, the fifth Misery, arises from habitual[119] fear of death and it is deep seated in the learned even. This fear fosters on itself. It too is born of ignorance because we are made to believe that we die. We have no first-hand experience of death; moreover, no one can have! We see death or change in other [drishya], but can never in Self [Drashtri or Knower].

As long as I am *knowing*, I am not dead. As regards not knowing, that is preposterous. ... The statement 'I am dead' is a lie. Life [or consciousness] just cannot be denied — DENIAL ITSELF CONFIRMS LIFE!

We are so accustomed to these Miseries that there is no moment when we do not take refuge in notions of permanence, purity, pleasure, and *me 'n' myness* (ego, person, and possessions). We bolster ourselves with possessions and identifications. We nurture attachment and aversion. Fear of death haunts us throughout our life, no matter how learned we are. We are so habitual of these

---

[117] In Yoga, bhoga (experience) is explained as disappearance of essential distinction between mind (sattva) and Self (Purusha). [III 35]

[118] All existence is indeed pain. [II 15]

[119] The word habitual is deliberately used to suggest that fear of death can be corrected.

Miseries that without them we perceive our being threatened. Just imagine: dreams and daydreams are our compulsions! We invest a lot of time in them. ... Our entire life personifies Kleshas!

Kleshas (Miseries) act as tributaries for the reservoir of past good and bad deeds or their impressions. As long as Kleshas are (or the root cause, Avidya is) there, there inevitably are shoots (consequences) in the form of rebirths, lives of different spans, and cyclic experiences of pleasure and pain.

Beware! Kleshas lure and trap unwise and unscrupulous!

CHAPTER THREE

The Avidya Sutra

THE FORMULA OF WISDOM

Recall or if necessary revisit Synopsis.

Perceiving or misjudging permanence, purity, pleasure (sukha), and Self (Atma) in what indeed is impermanent, impure, pain (duhkha), and non-self is called *Avidya* (*Ignorance of Reality*). [II 5]

First, we have a feel of traditional view on the sutra. Following is a close translation of commentary of Sage Vyasa:

Perception of permanence in impermanent effects is seen in expressions like: eternal is the Earth; eternal are the heavens along with Moon and stars; eternal are gods. [They in fact last far longer than our usual notions of time!]

Similar is the notion of purity (in impure and impious things); body gets filthy and loathsome [despite regular baths and ceremonial purifications]. As it is also said in verse:

The wise know body as impure for reasons of
Its location [in womb], its origin,
Its process of upkeep, perspiration, and death,
Moreover, as it needs regular cleaning.

— thus is purity believed by ignorant in what is impure.

The maiden looks charming like crescent Moon; her limbs as if made of honey and nectar; emerged as from Moon itself; large eyes emulating petals of blue lotus and sporting flashes; virtually rejuvenating this earthly (mortal) life ...

— thus what is attributed to what! Thus is nursed (false) notion of purity [beauty[120]] in what is impure. Similarly are explained notions of virtue in what is sin and of purpose in what is meaningless (vain). Moreover, about the notion of pleasure in what is pain is spoken as:

> For reasons of pain from change, anguish, and impressions and from conflicting guna-processes, all existence is indeed pain for a man of Viveka. [II 15]

— notion of pleasure there in what is pain is Avidya.

Similar is the notion of self in what is non-self. External accessories, whether animate or inanimate; body, the vehicle of experience; mind as instrument of Purusha (Self) — in any of these other-than-self manifestations, perception of Self is Avidya. It is also said:

> Believing as self anything manifest or else,
> He who revels in its growth as personal growth,
> And grieves at its ruin as personal loss –
> Such person is indeed fast asleep (unaware).

Avidya has four quarters.[121] It is the source of train of Kleshas (Miseries) and of the potent merit-demerit residuum (reservoir of impressions of past good and bad deeds).

Grammatically, Avidya should be understood as positive entity as in the case of amitra (a = no or absence, and mitra = friend). The compound word here means neither 'absence of friend' nor 'just friend' (so-called friend) but something [positive existent] contrary to friend, an enemy. ... So is Avidya neither right knowledge nor its absence, but another (positive) cognition, which is contrary to Vidya (Knowledge).

---

120 Which is either fleeting or personal (beholder-dependent)!

121 Those are rather misconceptions or paradoxes.

Suggestions, Predicates, and Paradoxes

Let us now analyse this cryptic sutra!

In its first impression, it looks ridiculous! It just talks about the obvious proposition. Something is not its negation! Yes, true, that is always the case.

Regarding impermanent as permanent et al is fallacious and illogical. So too regarding permanent as impermanent et al. BE CAREFUL! Second assertion is though equally fallacious but it goes against Avidya Sutra!

THEN, IS AVIDYA SUTRA MYSTIC DESPITE ITS DEFICIENCY? Perhaps, we have to trust its wisdom!

Definition of Avidya alerts us precisely against regarding impermanent as permanent, impure as pure, pain as pleasure, and non-self as self (but not vice versa). ...

To our relief and amazement, the definition will be found stunningly brilliant. ... It in fact takes us to the most trusted and practical guide (*guru*) for our redemption! This is so because we shall see in the next chapter that PERMANENCE, PURITY, PLEASURE, AND SELF (PERSONALITY) ARE PARADOXES OF LIFE. We cannot find any object in the world (Drishya) that could truly be called permanent, pure (virtuous or determinable), pleasure, or Self. ... However, it is initially difficult to swallow. Reader can get a clue to this in the universality of pain discussed in chapter 1.1 or yoga sutra II 15. Moreover, every object is an object of knowledge and therefore non-self (*i.e.*, other than me) in terms of Viveka. Therefore, even if objects or world were permanent, pure, and pleasure, it can be of no avail to Self (me)!

In other words, this whole WORLD (DRISHYA, SEEABLE) IS IMPERMANENT, IMPURE, PAIN, AND NON-SELF. Impermanent could be changing, transient, or short-lived; and impure signifies unclean, imperfect, immoral, elusive, or indeterminate. Impermanence, impurity, pain/suffering, and non-self are predicates or rather the **dharma** (law) of all objects and ideas.

The word AND used in the above postulate is crucial because by virtue of any single misconception (or paradox of life) Avidya sneaks in. Suppose someone believes world as only impure and impermanent, and accordingly acts immoral and kills others. He can say that he did not violate the law of things – by acting immoral [because there is nothing like pure or moral here] and by killing only impermanents (mortals)! However, his argument is flawed in terms of Avidya as a whole. He must have been prompted by sadistic pleasure and/or by selfish motives. In terms of Avidya, he is deluded because he nurses misconceptions of *pleasure* and *self* (person and property).

Superior Formula of Wisdom

In so-called incompleteness of Avidya [which had been our initial suspicion] lies hidden the precise nature of world. The Avidya Sutra when rightly understood remedies universal misery. Rather when we remember this much alone that ALL IS IMPERMANENT, IMPURE, PAIN, AND OTHER-THAN-SELF, we nip Avidya (and Kleshas) in the bud. For example, when all is understood as impermanent etc., then we *cannot* nurse notions of permanence etc. in whatsoever object. ... Avidya Sutra becomes a SUPERIOR ALTERNATIVE to Viveka (Seer-Seeable Distinction) and Purusha-khyati (knowledge of Self). ... It even obviates the knowledge of elaborate theories and skips such counts of 25 or 26 principles like Prakriti, intelligence, ego-sense, mind, senses, gross elements, and so on.

It is foolproof criterion! Without it we could be mistakenly claiming Seer-Seeable Distinction and still nursing conjunctions (identifications) as *I am sick or miserable, I have grown rich, I am humble and virtuous*, etc. ... It is truly potent in warding off Kleshas.

Besides, surrender becomes genuine and qualitative – because there is no ego, no person, and no property to identify with.

Likewise, mind and its processes become drishya (non-self), impure, subject to change, and painful and therefore fit to be inhibited.

This formula of wisdom is secular too.

Avidya Sutra is so revelatory, so encompassing, and still so simple to apply by everyone that Sage Patanjali did not feel it necessary to separately introduce and treat Vidya (knowledge) in his work[122].

The succinct formula couches many mystical phrases and admonitions within it, like: neti neti [*i.e.*, Truth or Self is neither this nor that]; the Buddhist Truths of Suffering and No-self[123]; theories of Advaita (non-dualism) and Maya [transitory, illusory, and elusive nature of world]; Know thyself; and 'I know nothing except the fact of my ignorance.'[124]

---

122 Separate treatment of Vidya and its precise determination were avoided – possibly for reasons of *aśuchi* (or the paradox of purity).

123 Here it fits well in the sense that (1) we cannot know Self objectively and (2) whatever we know or can know is non-self.

124 Last two were favourites of Socrates.

❧ Ominous Avidya ☙

My mother used to tell a story from The Mahabharata epic. Arjuna was a great archer of his times. He was also favourite cousin of Lord Krishna [who acted as his charioteer and preached The Bhagavad Gita on the battlefield].

Once the two cousins were going to river for morning bath when Arjuna joked to Lord Krishna, 'It is heard that you possess the so-called divine illusion-issuing power (Maya[125]) but you have never demonstrated the same to me!' Lord Krishna was amused and deferred reply for a suitable occasion. They reached the river. They walked into it and took the dip.

When Arjuna came up, he found himself smeared with mud and the riverbank looked deserted. He was possessed by the state. He suspected that the bank could have been like that before he entered! He could not recollect properly. ... To his embarrassment, he could not find his cousin even, nor the clothes that he had left there before taking dip. He reasoned to himself that Lord Krishna, who was well known for his pranks, must have disappeared with clothes! But he was not sure!

Then, far away in one direction, he saw dust rising in the sky. He saw chariots coming that side. King of the state appeared to be passing from there. Naked Arjuna hid himself behind the bushes.

While passing by, king's attendants noticed him hiding suspiciously behind bushes. They halted chariots to check who he was and what he was up to. However, their joy bore no bounds when they discovered him to be Arjuna. King called this success providential! ... In fact, for some devious

---

[125] Under its charm, human beings err.

act the king had been cursed to be a leper and was advised by soothsayers that in order to be delivered from ugly curse, he should trace Arjuna and make him marry his daughter. ...

To his bewilderment, Arjuna was given royal robes and taken to the capital. King's daughter was married to Arjuna. King had been delivered from the curse. Time passed by happily for the royal couple.

Then, as fate had willed it, Arjuna's charming companion passed away. Arjuna felt immensely grieved, and in dire gloom decided to end his life on the funeral pyre of his wife. The king tried to pacify him and even offered him for marriage his younger daughter who was equally charming. However, this did not assuage Arjuna. ...

At that moment, Lord Krishna appeared to rescue Arjuna saying, 'Let us go – I have finished my bath.' With this ended his nightmare, a tumble of Maya!

So how far our experiences can be actual! Avidya strikes all of us every moment; for we are unaware and unwary! According to philosopher Shankara, for individuals whether awake or asleep, Avidya keeps projecting worlds of experience and alluring individuals. Everything deludes as real and meaningful! [Appendix B]

Avidya therefore should rightly become for all target of apprehension. Four paradoxes, which we elaborate in the next chapter, act as its haven.

CHAPTER FOUR

Paradoxes of Life

❄

PERMANENCE, PURITY, PLEASURE, PERSONALITY

Permanence

> Everything flows and nothing stays...
> You can't step twice into the same river. (*Heraclitus*)

River is flowing every moment; much water flows down the stream by the time you put next step into the river.

Things of course are undergoing change, but belief in constancy of things is comforting! Misconception of permanence and eternity of objects lurks. We remain greedy about higher status, power, and possessions in the expectation that they last and stand by us forever!

Our fortunes wane; our resources dwindle; and limitless universe around is in a state of flux. With the help of accurate scientific instruments we can detect imperceptible and infinitesimally small changes or movements, *e.g.*, drifting continents, growing (forming) mountain ranges, etc. ...

Even what is not changing is susceptible to change! ...

Nevertheless, we overlook impermanence. ... So many historical names and long-standing institutions give a semblance of constancy to the world! ...

Even otherwise, we fear that change can open up innumerable possibilities – unpleasant and dreadful. We do not feel secure with change. Notion of permanence in what indeed is impermanent comforts us, even if its stint is short. ... Ultimately, we are bound to feel frustrated and dejected.

Thus, we need to be consciously aware of transience all around and not nurture Avidya (or misery) any longer.

Purity

Somewhere melodies escape lutes;
Somewhere heart-rending mournful wails;
Somewhere scholars engage in dialectics;
Somewhere drunkards take up brawl;
Somewhere charming maidens arouse our passion;
Somewhere loathing physique worn out by age;
I do not know if this world is a tonic or toxic! (*Bhartrihari*)

Nothing is either good or bad,
but thinking makes it so. (*W. Shakespeare*)

Unlike impermanence of things, impurity is perceptional in origin and even independent of things themselves. Impurity signifies imperfect, immoral, indeterminate, or elusive character of objects or ideas – due to our *changing* mind, values, and judgements.

Things are impure. They may not be precisely as or the way we see them. For example, what we call virtue and morality generally turns out to be serving our own interest and greed![126] ... What is beauty? The answer remains quiet subjective; it solely rests on the beholder. ... When greeted with the question, 'How are you?' the reply is rarely true or absolute. It depends on how 'you' fare in *comparison/relation* to others. Or, one may not reveal true feelings and emotions.

Every experience *by itself* becomes difficult to be named *e.g.* pleasure or pain! Look at the line drawn in the box below. Is it long or short? Neither. By itself, length of line is just meaningless. It is long if you draw a shorter line along it or if you are used to seeing shorter lines; and short otherwise.

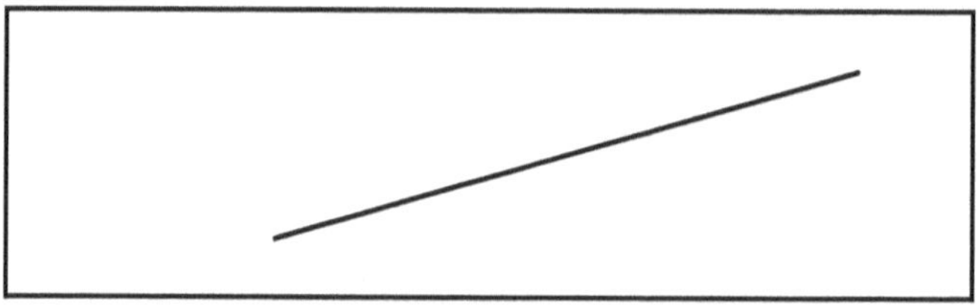

NEITHER-LONG-NOR-SHORT LINE

What is more, impurity is pervasive. *Nothing* is pure – whether at physical level as clean, hygienic, or pollution-free; or figuratively as virtuous, righteous, moral, honest, or just!

Nevertheless, it is not the intention of Yoga that we should abandon it (being unachievable or indeterminate). It ought to be an IDEAL TO BE EVER STRIVED FOR. Obstinate claim of one's purity and blanket disapproval of others' viewpoints will be unaccommodating and unprogressive. Such attitude can expose us to diseases, vices, sins, conflicts, and immoralities. Complacency about purity should be carefully avoided. ...

---

[126] Possibly that is why *all* undertakings (works) are said to be shrouded in demerit or instigated by Avidya. [*Cf.* BG XVIII 48 and Appendix B.]

Possibly, that is what *purity of mind* in Yoga is! [*Cf.* YS II 41.] It is otherwise mistaken for nursing and acting out good thoughts. But we regress to the same problem: indeterminate nature of things, or here the DEFINITION OF GOOD! Good or moral is difficult to be *commonly* determined and accepted. It will vary and even conflict among different societies – given their preferred beliefs, customs, and backgrounds. Killings in war may be genocide for the victimised or at-risk society, but heroic for the killers or gainers. Not only that, within one society too, individual morality (standpoint) could vary from that of society or majority![127] ...

Purity of mind lies in putting a constant question mark on own opinions, assumptions, and hypotheses, while keeping in perspective the others'.[128] Otherwise, we are putting final labels on elusive and indeterminable things and situations!

DO NOT ASSUME AN AIR OF CLEAR-CUT FINALITY!

---

[127] What is morality in any given time or place? It is what the majority then and there happen to like and immorality is what they dislike. (Alfred North Whitehead) *Liking is an arbitrary and fragile basis for morality!*

[128] The unexamined life is not worth living. (Socrates)

Pleasure (Sukha)

All is indeed pain to Vivekin (man of Viveka). [II 15]

We discussed about pain in chapter 1.1. Reader was cautioned there not to take it pessimistically.

One suspicion can still lurk in the mind of reader. If *all* is pain, then how can yoga provide remedy?

However, it provides – some explanations are given below:

- The word ALL cannot include Seer Self (Drashtri), being unseeable/unknowable.
- RECALL PREVIOUS PARADOXES and peep into the nature of pleasure in their light. In this world of impermanence and impurity, pleasure in any form too ought to be transitory and impure (painful)! ...
- Paradox of pleasure afflicts us because generally for us SUPPLY OF PLEASURE IS NEVER ENOUGH AND CONSTANT. Our expectation and greed for pleasure make even the available pleasure disappointing. ... Yoga simply breaks our fixation on pleasure, which makes us daydream, fantasise, and miss the present. Pleasure becomes no less than mind game, a wild goose chase! Pleasure is pain unless paradox of pleasure is exposed.
- Pleasure like pain stems from OTHER (DRISHYA), which according to Yoga has *relative or subjective existence*[129]. Therefore, how can we be sure of its constant supply? In addition, other (non-self) has nothing to do with Self in terms of Viveka!
- Furthermore, our fixation on pleasure creates a fictitious and anomalous DIVIDE within the observable world (Drishya) – some things are seen as pleasure

---

[129] YS II 21

and others as pain. Yoga does not approve any division other than Viveka.[130] Divisions other than Drashtri-Drishya are figment of mind!

- Pleasure and pain are PERSPECTIVES, which keep alternating[131]. Even something exotic and glamorous can look ordinary after a while. There is nothing like absolute or universal pleasure.
- Pleasure and pain are RELATIVE terms; neither exists independent of other.
- What is said as PAIN TO YOGI (vivekin) above appears to be enigmatic! Yogi and pain are incompatible. If yogi too has to suffer, then what is the charm in pursuing yoga? However, it is not like that. It can be explained like this:
  - Yogi sees all this as non-self (drishya) and distinct from himself (Self). Therefore, he sees no purpose to be served by it. He is rather liberated from pain! [Pain arises from non-self.]
  - Yogi [having outgrown his ego bounds] shall be pained to see ignorance, injustice, and inequity in practice all around and will be filled with compassion over what people are not sharing in life due to Avidya. I am reminded of a lyric of Hindi film *Anand* (or ananda) revealing such mysterious concern:

    A sweet puzzle it is;
    Own mind turns foe;
    Being mine still
    Shares others' woe ...
    Whenever far-away Sun sets
    And evening bride shyly sneaks in ...

Yogi suffers (or seems to suffer) because others are *no more other* to him!

---

130 'ekam eva ḍarśanam khyāṭir eva ḍarśanam,' thus Sage Vyasa in his commentary on YS I 3 quotes an ancient teacher.

131 Phenomenon of *changing* mind supplies the crucial justification for paradoxes of purity and pleasure.

Personality (Assumed Self)

This ambition I have realised and this I will realise in time;
This much wealth I already possess and more too would be mine.

I slayed this enemy and tomorrow others too get slayed.
I have become lord, enjoyer, almighty, and gratified. [BG XVI 13-14]

In ignorance, personality is perceived as Self. Personality is indeed evanescent, notional Self – a substitute that works with ever newer, changing masks for a long time. The most commonly used word 'I' remains most widely misunderstood. In ignorance, we use language of impermanence and change in describing Self.

We do not know Self but only personality and property – which unfortunately remain just knowable (drishya; or objects of knowledge or of Self) and therefore non-self. … Paradox of person is the most complex and challenging one among all the paradoxes.

We identify ourselves [or our Self] with non-self objects and attributes. The range of non-self is quite extensive and encompassing. It includes even:

'All external accessories (objects or beings serving as extensions or aids); the physical body and its organs (*viz.* senses), which help in experiencing the world; and the mind and intellect.

'To look upon anything manifest or unmanifest as self and then to revel in its growth as personal growth and to grieve at its ruin as one's personal failure — all this is nescience, ignorance.'[132] [Refer to Sage Vyasa's commentary in chapter 5.3.]

---

[132] Drashtri (Seer Self) is *just knowing* (Consciousness) which though pure resembles (or is identified with) the contents or objects (thoughts etc.) of mind. [II 20]

What do we learn from previous paradoxes? Every concept of Self will be impermanent, impure, and painful. This blend with non-self objects and attributes would remain transitory, elusive, and painful (frustrating).

The Upanishads have brilliantly admonished us with the words NETI NETI (meaning neither this nor that). Façade of Self is quite alluring and intriguing! Carefully separate non-self from knowledge of Self. Say no-no!

DISTINGUISH YOURSELF FROM THE FOUR PARADOXES!

SECTION SIX

Self (Atman)

UNDENIABLE & INDESCRIBABLE

Seer Self (Drashtri) is just unseeable (a-drishya).[133]

Consciousness abides; personality fades/phases out.

CHAPTERS

133 This is what Viveka means. Moreover, according to Avidya Sutra, Seeable (Drishya, world) is … non-self.

> This Self — being nearer and more intimate — is dearer than son; dearer than wealth; dearer than everything else. He who warns someone holding non-self objects as dear, like 'Your dear might perish and make you cry!' is indeed a prophet — it will happen like that.
>
> Therefore, Self alone should be meditated as dear. He who holds Self alone as dear, his dear ones will not perish or desert him. [BU I iv 8]

A single crisis can demolish our notions of self. None of sons, wealth, and the rest is dear or indeed stands by us. ... Even we can forsake them for self-sake.

Every imaginable object is an object of or exists in relation to Self and therefore fit to be regarded as *other* (non-self) and *parartha* (relative existence; not existing by itself or for its own sake). In short, everything exists for the sake of Self. [II 21]

Meditate on Yoga phrase FOR THE SAKE OF SELF (***svartha***) in order to realise Self.[134] Generally, we take svartha in the narrow sense, *viz.* self-interest, selfishness, and greed. However, Yoga uses its profound sense, *viz.* SELF-EXISTENCE (absolute existence; existing by itself or for its own sake) and WELFARE OF ALL.[135] ...

Either way, awareness of svartha rewards devotee with knowledge of and establishment in Self.

Accordingly, we take up *selfishness, self-existent, non-self,* and *all* in the following chapters. Last chapter of this section is consummatory.

---

134 स्वार्थसंयमात् पुरुषज्ञानम्। (svārṭhasaṃyamāṭ puruṣajñānam.) [III 35]

135 Sva (self, own) indeed signifies (1) Universal Self and (2) universe as self. Recall svadhyaya also.

CHAPTER ONE

Selfishness

YAJÑA

Meditate on Yoga phrase 'for the sake of Self' (svartha) as already said.

> Spouse is not dear for the sake of spouse;
> But for one's own sake!
> Sons are not dear for the sake of sons;
> But for one's own sake!
> Wealth is not dear for the sake of wealth;
> But for one's own sake!
> Not all is dear for the sake of all;
> But for one's own sake![136]

Selfishness, greed, and covetousness lie at the root of our thought processes and their execution. WE NEVER OBLIGE ANYBODY! No work or service to please others is undertaken without the prospect of personal benefit or satisfaction! We even twist virtue and morality to suit and serve own/personal purpose.[137] ALL UNDERTAKINGS ARE SELFISH; we tell lie if we say we did it for others. The Gita regards all undertakings as enveloped in demerit, like fire in smoke. [BG XVIII 48] Philosopher Shankara explains all works and

---

136 आत्मनस्तु कामाय सर्वं प्रियं भवति। (āṭmanas ṭu kāmāya sarvam priyam bhavaṭi.) [BU II iv 5]

137 The primary and sole foundation of virtue or of the proper conduct in life is to seek our own profit. (Spinoza)

their accessories as instigated by Avidya (Ignorance of Reality). [Appendix B]

Yoga too is critical of selfishness because the ultimate state of yoga is described as 'freedom from selfish motives.'[138]

There is merit in this cynicism. But what is the remedy for this ubiquitous selfishness? How can we escape this?

It is NOT POSSIBLE TILL our personal welfare remains primary, central to the welfare of all! NOT POSSIBLE TILL we do not know Self! Without knowing Self, we cannot be truly selfish! Without that, we confuse Self with personality, become selfish, and serve personality [false self].[139] … AVIDYA REMAINS THE ORIGINAL SIN!

Scriptures extol concepts of sacrifice (**yajña**[140] – general welfare or charity for the sake/benefit of all) and of duty (**dharma**) and enjoin charitable works as one's solemn duty. Unfortunately, selfishness defiles every charity. [BG III 9-16 *passim.*]

> All works but for yajña (sacrifice) verily bind and taint. …
>
> When in the beginning, Lord of Creatures (Prajapati)
> Created mankind with yajña, He enjoined:
> Ye prosper with it! It will fulfil your wishes!
> For ye thus foster macrocosmic gods,
> Who in turn foster ye through law of cyclic welfare. …
>
> But one who does not foster them in return (through yajña)
> Breaches this wheel of sacrifice;
> Leads verily a life of thief — purposeless and sinful. …
>
> Virtuous are ones who enjoy

---

[138] puruṣārṭhaśūnya [IV 34]

[139] Alternatively, selfishness stems from aviveka or Samyoga (Drashtri-Drishya Conjunction) in the sense that whatever we know as Self is indeed knowable (drishya) and therefore erroneous (in terms of Viveka). To do anything for such self is frustrating!

[140] यज्ञार्थात्कर्मणोऽन्यत्र लोकोऽयं कर्मबन्धनः। (yajñārṭhāṭ karmaṇo'nyaṭra loko'yam karmabanḍhanaḥ.)

The left-over of distributes of sacrifice;
While sinful undertake sacrifice
Primarily for themselves.[141]

In other words, selfishness is repugnant to yajña (general welfare). Our *primary* motive decides the nature of our acts and their outcomes. WHERE THERE IS SELFISHNESS OR GREED[142], THERE CAN BE NO YAJÑA AND NO COMMON WELFARE.[143] In selfishness, we are too obsessed to give, and we tend to tilt give-and-take balance in our favour.

In Avidya or in selfishness, even yajña is sin. No sacrifice (yajña) without self-sacrifice!

So too in the admonition 'In surrender to Him, enjoy!' [chapter 4.2], surrender takes precedence over selfishness. Enjoyment naturally flows from surrender.

Virtuous and blessed are those who do not nurture this illusion of selfishness. Their actions promote nothing but common welfare. In that collective welfare, they enjoy their lot (the residue of yajña). This seems paradoxical, but this is the law – sacrifice yourself [do not nurture illusory selfishness] and enjoy!

My mother tells another story from The Puranas (Hindu mythology). Once Narada, bard of heavens, felt conceited – no other devotee in all the worlds can rival his devotion to Lord Vishnu and his position alongside the Lord. Lord Vishnu endowed with surpassing grace wanted to reprove him.

Lord called Narada and confessed to him His secret desire to taste flesh of His dearest devotee. Narada was

---

141 यज्ञशिष्टाशिनः सन्तो मुच्यन्ते सर्वकिल्बिषैः।
भुञ्जते ते त्वघं पापा ये पचन्त्यात्मकारणात्॥
(yajñaśiṣṭāśinaḥ sanṭo muchyanṭe sarvakilbiṣāiḥ; bhuñjaṭe ṭe ṭvagham pāpā ye pachanṭyāṭmakāraṇāṭ.)

142 Greed is tamas (being ignorance) and rajas (when acted on).

143 बुभुक्षितः किं न करोति पापम्। (bubhukṣiṭaḥ kim na karoṭi pāpam.) What kind of immorality a greedy person does not commit!

stupefied with this *holy* desire! Still, submissively he picked weighing scales in one hand and his lute in the other and proceeded on his mission to worlds, in search of Lord's dearest devotee and to obtain his flesh if possible.

Narada announced in the worlds and invited devotees to offer their flesh for Lord. People became paranoid to hear this unusual desire.

Nevertheless, one devotee came forward. He was a skinny skeleton, too emaciated by austere life. He himself started scraping his flesh and putting in the scales, but was disappointed to find that it was not going to be enough. Narada despaired but devotee did not want to miss this opportunity to please the Lord. The devotee then popped into the scales so that his whole person could make up for the divine feast. Shortfall was conspicuous! ... Narada still decided to take him seated in scales, to heavens. On seeing all this, Lord Vishnu smiled to the devotee in approval! ... Narada realised his folly – why he went in search of the dearest devotee; he could have promptly offered himself to Lord!

DEVOTION AND SURRENDER DEMAND GENUINE READINESS FOR SELF-SACRIFICE.
THERE LIES THE HIGHEST MERIT!

CHAPTER TWO

Self-existent

❄

SVAYAMBHU

ॐ

Mystical Syllable *Om*

[Teacher-Disciple Dialogue of Appendix B provides crucial supplementary reading for this chapter.]

Whatever we know or can know is not Self. In other words, Self is not knowable (*i.e.*, adrishya). Self will remain unseeable, indescribable.[144] But isn't it agnostic?

> There is a story[145] about Chuang Tzu, a master sage from China. One day he woke up with an intriguing puzzle. He would not leave it until satisfied. When disciples saw master in fix, they thronged him in disbelief and service and asked him what disturbed his calm. The master explained to them that in dream he saw himself as butterfly, flitting about flowers in a garden. Disciples could not believe that such routine dream could perturb their master. For them it was master's prank; there was no worth in complaining about dreams.

---

144 The Bhagavad Gita calls Self as achinṭya (unthinkable) and aprameya (indefinable). [BG II 18, 25]

145 It was told by Osho during his discourses on Lord Krishna.

Nonetheless, disciples tried to divert his attention, calling all that quite normal. On the contrary, for the intelligent master, his identity was at stake – whether he was Chuang Tzu [dreaming of butterfly at night] or butterfly [dreaming of Chuang Tzu during day]! ...

This IDENTITY CRISIS looms large for all of us, though overlooked! Who am I? Puzzle of the above story is deliberate and insightful. It shatters all our notions of Self and, side by side, verity of waking and dream states.[146] ... Experiences of either state are negated in the other. While awake, dream is false; and in dream, waking is meaningless [false]!

Our identity or personality is altogether blown when we take into account the mental process **sleep** (dreamless sleep[147]). According to Yoga, dreamless sleep rests on the notion of non-existence or nothingness. [I 10] We *mentally* experience nothingness. The state is also called perfect slumber where one does not yearn for any desire whatsoever, nor sees any dream whatsoever. [MU 5]

> Here [in deep sleep] father is no more father; mother no more mother; worlds no more worlds; gods no more gods; The Vedas no more Vedas. Here thief is no more a thief; murderer no more a murderer; low caste no more a low caste; labourer no more a labourer; ascetic no more an ascetic — [here Sleeper is] followed by neither virtue nor vice for he [for the time being] goes beyond all mental sorrows [born of duality]. [BU IV iii 22]

Here all our identities of waking and dream states, whether Chuang Tzu or butterfly, fail us – no matter if duration of sleep is brief. Understandably, our identity ought to be void-like and not determinable extrinsically![148]

---

146 In Hymn to Mind in chapter 3.1, mind was described as roaming places near and far, while awake and in dreams.

147 Non-REM (rapid eye movement) phase of sleep

148 Yoga is careful in describing Samadhi as 'as if devoid of Self.' Self is void-like but not void. Self is undeniable, still indescribable.

[Had there been no dream and sleep states, the world (Drishya) would have been impossible to repudiate and transcend!]

Had light been conscious like us, it would have believed itself rich on lighting prized objects, and poor on lighting commonplace objects. Not only that, on lighting nothing or an empty room, it would have experienced a sense of loss of identity as we experience in sleep.

Light is neither of objects illumined and unillumined, but quite distinct, LIGHT — THAT ILLUMINES OBJECTS. So too, Self (Consciousness) is distinct from or unaffected by possible objects of consciousness. [Different terms used for consciousness do not matter a bit.]

Experiences, information, and knowledge of waking and dream states *cannot* determine our identity.

> In the three states, name or imagine any object —
> Experiencer, experience, or experienced;
> Discrete from states/roles stay I (Self) —
> Just conscious, witness, and ever shiva.[149]

We indeed are pure, unattached [unqualified]. We seemingly roam between the two ends (waking and dream) like fish between two banks; and indulge in the objects there. WE ACCRUE NOTHING, OWN NOTHING, AND OWE NOTHING![150]

---

149 त्रिषु धामसु यद्भोग्यं भोक्ता भोगश्च यद्भवेत्।
तेभ्यो विलक्षणः साक्षी चिन्मात्रोऽहं सदा शिवः॥
(ṭriṣu ḍhāmasu yaḍbhogyam bhokṭā bhogaścha yaḍbhaveṭ;
ṭebhyo vilakṣaṇaḥ sākṣī chinmāṭro'ham saḍā śivaḥ) [KVU 18]

150 स वा एष एतस्मिन्स्वप्ने रत्वा चरित्वा दृष्ट्वैव पुण्यं च पापं च पुनः प्रतिन्यायं प्रतियोन्याद्रवति बुद्धान्तायैव। स यत्तत्र किञ्चित्पश्यत्यनन्वागतस्तेन भवति। असङ्गो ह्ययं पुरुष इति। (sa vā eṣa eṭasmin svapne raṭvā chariṭvā ḍṛṣtvāiva puṇyam cha pāpam cha punaḥ praṭinyāyam praṭiyonyāḍravaṭi buḍḍhānṭāiva. sa yaṭṭaṭra kiñchiṭpaśyaṭyananvāgaṭas ṭena sa bhavaṭi. asaňgo hyayam puruṣa iṭi.) [*Cf.* BU IV iii 15-16 and YS II 20.]

The Mandukya Upanishad reveals a mysterious relationship between three constituent letters of ॐ (Om) and the three states (*i.e.*, waking, dream, and sleep). Three letters a, u, m correspond to the three roles of individual, namely: Waker [outward-wise], Dreamer [inward-wise], and Sleeper [neither-wise].[151] The Upanishad declares:

> Nonetheless, beyond letters, words, and concepts and beyond [distinct from] phenomena [states, experiences, and roles — *Drishya*] is the Fourth, Auspicious, One, Omkar — verily the Self of all.[152]

The mystical syllable Om (ॐ) and its chant (Omkar) provide us true perspective! ...

SELF IS DISCRETE FROM PHENOMENA (DRISHYA) AND STILL SELF OF ALL!

---

[151] Terms waker, dreamer, and sleeper were used by Sri Aurobindo for the three roles of individual.

[152] अमात्रश्चतुर्थोऽव्यवहार्यः प्रपञ्चोपशमः शिवोऽद्वैत एवमोङ्कार आत्मैव। (amāṭraśchaṭurṭho'vyavahāryaḥ prapañchopaśamaḥ śivo'ḍvāiṭa evam oṅkāra āṭmāiva.) [MU 12]

Consciousness

Now in the light of discussion so far, recall yoga phrase *svartha* and search for what fits this criterion. ...

CONSCIOUSNESS EXISTS for its own sake or irrespective of others. It is self-evident (self-intimating) and therefore undeniable. It is self-existent (*svartha*)!

All known or knowable objects depend upon consciousness for their manifestation [existence]. *For us,* other objects exist so long as, to the extent, and the way we are aware of them; they do not exist in unawareness. ... Therefore, NOTHING OTHER THAN CONSCIOUSNESS EXISTS.

Consciousness itself exists *absolutely*; all else relatively. Furthermore, it alone can be expected to be true, independent bliss (bliss-in-itself); else being illusory. We have thus arrived at the triune principle sat-chit-ananda

EXISTENCE = CONSCIOUSNESS = BLISS

As a rule of thumb, remember first three letters of English alphabet. Recite A-B-C loud; intone it. A stands for **a**nanda (bliss), B for 'to **b**e (exist),' and C for 'to **s**ee (be **c**onscious).' Letters represent the nature of Universal Self (Brahma or Purusha).

In Yoga terminology, the equation can be rephrased as Drashtri (Seer), who is just knowing[153] (*i.e.*, consciousness), is self-existent (svartha). [II 20, III 35] Drashtri enjoys the state of Kaivalya (blissful aloneness) which is described as escape/liberation from painful world, or as establishment in Self. [II 25, IV 34]

---

[153] YS II 20

Negation

Admonition 'Net neti' meaning 'neither this nor that' is remarkable. Use it in anyway. Rest assured – only knowable (drishya) is going to be repudiated. You will be established in Self even if you do not know what Drashtri (Self) is! ... Self is non-negatable.

Philosopher Shankara derived from negation interesting positive statements about Consciousness [Self].[154] He analyses types of negation and then infers about the non-negatable. For example, **absence** is a form of negation. 'Something is absent somewhere' can be rephrased, as 'that something is *not* at the said place.' Now this negation 'absence somewhere' cannot fit with non-negatable consciousness. So consciousness is 'non-absent anywhere' or, in other words, OMNIPRESENT.

Similarly, 'absence during some period of time' implies 'something does/did/will *not* exist during said period of time.' This absence too cannot be predicated to consciousness. Consciousness therefore exists throughout time; or is ETERNAL (without beginning and without end).

Negation also arises from **difference** due to change over time or from distinguishing characteristics. For example, when we say 'A changes into B with time,' it simply means 'A will *not* remain the same over time.' Negation of any such difference in consciousness suggests: consciousness is CHANGELESS. Similarly, difference due to distinguishing characteristics can be phrased as 'A is *not* B.' Negation of such difference in consciousness would mean: there are no differences or no different classes in consciousness; or consciousness is ONLY ONE OF ITS KIND.

Consciousness [Self] is thus concluded by philosopher Shankara as the only reality, eternal, omnipresent, and timeless.

---

[154] Refer to 'Indian Philosophy' in Encyclopaedia Britannica.

In terms of Avidya Sutra, predicates of world (Drishya) are impermanent, impure, pain, and non-self. But can we infer something about Drashtri? Yes.

We have already noted that Drashtri is 'just seeing' (consciousness) and is blissful – being 'established in Self' or 'liberated from pain.' Further, adjectives used by Yoga, namely: changeless[155] and pure[156] are also noteworthy.

Therefore, what holds true for Drishya, opposite holds for Drashtri.

DRASHTRI IS ETERNAL (PERMANENT), PURE, BLISS, AND TRUE SELF.

Our body, mind, ideas, and circumstances – all change drastically over time – from birth to adulthood, to old age. Personality fades, but our true identity [self-existent, self-evident consciousness] lingers as evidenced in such expressions as 'I am the same, so-and-so; you don't recognise me!'

Let us conclude with Sage Vyasa's comment on YS I 2:

> Unlike mind [which is drishya[157]], Power of Consciousness (Chiti) does not change; it does not move from object to object, rather objects are shown to it; it is pure and infinite.

---

[155]YS IV 18
[156] YS II 20
[157] YS IV 19

CHAPTER THREE

Non-self Drishya

THING OR THINK!

Reader will be intrigued to accept this chapter in the section Self. Drashtri and Drishya are just opposite; this is what Viveka means!

Through the Thou a person becomes I. (*Martin Buber*)

This chapter is intended to bring out Drishya (non-self) in all its aspects so that a comprehensive reflection of Self could be had. We here intend to approach Self through non-self or extended Self.

Parartha

We are familiar with Drishya (world) from the very first chapter. We revisit it with further evidence and with a better focus – after all we are approaching end of the book.

> Drishya (world; or all knowable) has: [1] **inherent conflict** due to three fundamental attributes (*gunas*[158]): *sattva* (light, virtue, and knowledge), *rajas* (motion, desire, passion, greed, and anger), and *tamas* (mass, inertia, vice, and ignorance); [2] assumes form of physical elements, senses (and mind), and self [ego]; and [3] provides experience (bhoga) to the ignorant and liberation (apavarga) to the realised.
>
> Drishya is Parartha. It exists for the sake of or relative to Drashtri (Self) and not itself. [II 18,21]

However, following propositions further augment and enrich our perspective of world.

> Transitory world is composed of waking and dream experiences, alluring[159] individuals, by virtue of Avidya. [Appendix B]
>
> Meditate all this knowable (Drishya) as impermanent, impure (elusive), pain, and non-self; to behave otherwise is repugnant to Avidya Sutra [II 5].

It is difficult to completely translate word *drishya* into English. It is translated as scene. However, it literally stands for seeable or knowable – whatever is known or can be known as an object or concept. In this sense, Drishya comprises whole of *observable* universe. It also includes my possessions, senses, and mind. ... All these are non-self (seeable) and not Seer Self (true me)!

In terms of Parartha, WORLD DOES NOT EXIST ABSOLUTELY; it depends upon consciousness for its manifestation. It

---

158 Words used for three attributes are prakāśa (light), kriyā (activity), and sṭhiṭi (stasis), respectively.

159 Experiences delude as real and meaningful.

changes in itself and also in our perceptions of it. That is why sometimes it pleases, sometimes irritates, and sometimes deludes. Thus world appears MULTI-FACETED [due to variety of perceptions] and not one. Understandably, such world disappears for the realised, while for others it continues to operate as constant and common proposition.[160]

For those who do not understand this nature of relative or illusory existence of world are unable to maintain distinction with objects and thoughts. Thoughts are confused with absolute truths; objects with Self [me]; and false agency (kartritva, doership) is superimposed on witness Self. In Yoga, this phenomenon is called BHOGA (experience). One who falls into error of bhoga keeps seeking identity and self-fulfilment in outside world (non-self). Remember: in bhoga, world (seeable) assumes form of Self (Seer).[161] [Bhoga is failure of Viveka.]

THIS WORLD RESTS ON KNOWLEDGE OR EXISTS IN MIND. However there is one problem with our knowledge [as already seen in chapter 3.2] – it is not foolproof and accordingly our whole edifice of knowledge would collapse! [Reader may also recall the paradox of purity of chapter 5.4.]

Not only that, if we can err once, we are susceptible to error anytime and anywhere (waking or dream). If rope-snake, mirage-water, and dreams [by virtue of their existence in mind or as knowledge] can fool us as real, then other assumptions and experiences of waking and dream states, which can not be acquired in any different way, too ought not to be valid! [Appendix B] ... This explains WORLD AS PRODUCT OF AVIDYA AND COMPRISING OF WAKING AND DREAM EXPERIENCES. It looks real and meaningful in ignorance.

'All that we see or seem is nothing but a dream within a dream.' (Edgar Allan Poe)

ISN'T WORLD A WAKING DREAM?

---

[160] *Cf.* YS II 22.

[161] Note the word āṭmaka in the definition of Drishya [II 18].

Now we scrutinise the three attributes (which constitute the effective cause of this universe). These too resolve the mystery of world. The three attributes (sattva, rajas, and tamas) can be seen as light, motion, and mass, respectively – which sound like popular terms of modern physics.

However, when these attributes are seen as knowledge, greed, and ignorance, remedy lies in subduing rajas and tamas. Every being in this world has these attributes but different proportions at different times. Generally, compared to sattva, proportion/dominance of rajas and tamas is high. We saw in chapter 3.1 that:

> Mind influenced by rajas and tamas loves power and possessions. When tamas dominates, mind is drawn to or is greedy about vice, ignorance, attachment, and helplessness. With tamas subsided, mind is still drawn [due to excess of rajas] but now to virtue, knowledge, detachment, and power, respectively. When rajas [too] subsides, mind is established in its being (sattva, illumination), revealing simply Discrimination (Viveka). And mind approaches Bounty-of-Virtue Samadhi, which is synonymous with Highest Knowledge.[162]

Therefore, SUBDUE RAJAS (GREED AND RESTLESS EFFORT) AND TAMAS (IGNORANCE AND SLOTH) WITH KNOWLEDGE AND REASON – otherwise, you seek non-self only. [Yamas, Niyamas, Asanas, and Pranayama eventually help in overcoming rajas and tamas; and side by side awaken awareness.]

There exists a CONNECTION BETWEEN THE THREE ATTRIBUTES AND THE THREE STATES. That is worth meditating. This is revealed in a traditional commentary on YS I 38. When rajas (activity) overpowers, it is waking state; when tamas dominates rajas, it is dream state; and when tamas completely overpowers rajas, it is dreamless sleep. Objects disappear in [dreamless] sleep state out of tamas (ignorance). Sattva is to be non-judgemental witness in the three states.

---

162 Commentary of Sage Vyasa on YS I 2

OBJECTS DISAPPEAR FOR A MAN OF VIVEKA IN ALL THREE STATES[163]. They are appearances [unreal]; they disappear in knowledge. ... So it is not strange if we call world a waking dream!

In terms of Avidya Sutra, world was seen as impermanent, impure, pain, and non-self. It is transitory, elusive, and perplexing. That too confirms world's illusory nature.

Experiences that are so real today over time get faded in memory and are no different from dreams! So how can those be called real at first experience too? ... This can be generalised to all experiences!

> Know this [world] as long [alluring] dream,
> Alternatively, an extended mental indulgence![164]

❋

163 *Cf.* YS II 22.

164 दीर्घस्वप्नमिमं विद्धि दीर्घं वा चित्तविभ्रमम्। (ḍīrghasvapnam imam viḍḍhi ḍīrgham vā chiṭṭavibhramam) [commentator Vijñānabhikṣu]

CHAPTER FOUR

I Am Brahma

❄

SAMBHUTI

One established in yoga can now appreciate this becoming or extension. Chapter is exceptional in nature. Excerpts in original appear in Appendix D.

> In the beginning, it was verily Brahma alone. He knew Himself only as 'I am Brahma (Boundless, All).'[165] Thence He became all this.
>
> Whosoever among gods appreciated this, he too became That. Likewise happened with sages and with humans. Him alone knowing all this, Sage Vamadeva proclaimed, 'I was Manu (the first man) and Surya (Sun).'
>
> The same holds valid even now; he who knows thus — 'I am Brahma' — realises all this. No gods ever can use such man as their subject. For he happens to be their Self too.
>
> However, he who regards divinity as separate from himself *viz.* 'He is else and me else' does not know indeed. As animal is to men, so is he to gods. [BU I iv10]

---

165 Drishya (world; knowable) rests on Drashtri (Knower) for its manifestation [existence].

I am Brahma (Boundless, All). I extend impartially and behave impartially to all — there is nothing like not-me or not-mine![166]

WHOLE WORLD IS FAMILY AND FAIRNESS BECOMES MY CONVICTION. FRIEND-FOE AND OWN-ALIEN DISTINCTIONS SIMPLY DROP.[167]

There remains NO SPECIFIC PURPOSE TO BE ACHIEVED! [IV 34] Moreover, purpose is a perception and transitory. This is establishment in Self or yoga. *Finis.*

---

166 All is Self here! Is it contrary to Viveka in the sense that Drishya (non-self) is seen as Self? No. In observing Viveka, obscurity between Self and non-self requires to be carefully avoided. But here that obscurity is simply precluded (for there is nothing like non-self).

167 अयं निजः परो वेति गणना लघुचेतसाम्। उदारचरितानां तु वसुधैव कुटुम्बकम्॥
(ayam nijaḥ paro veṭi gaṇanā laghucheṭasām; uḍāracharitānām ṭu vasuḍhāiva kutumbakam.)
Someone is my kin or stranger — thus calculate the narrow-minded. For liberal-minded, whole world is their family.

APPENDICES

APPENDIX A

Glossary

Italic words/names appear as separate entries. Transliteration hints[168] where necessary are provided in parentheses immediately after the entry.

Abhinivesha (-śa): fifth *klesha* described as yearning for life (or fear of death) — it is habitual in nature

Adrishya (a-ḍṛśya): non-*drishya* [unknowable *Purusha*]

Advaita (aḍvāiṭa): (1) non-duality (2) monistic Hindu philosophy

Ahimsa (ahiṃsā; not harming life): first *yama* that forbids violence, ill will, and malevolence

Ananda (ānanḍa): intrinsic bliss [unlike extrinsic pleasure (*sukha*) and pain (*duhkha*)]

Aparigraha: fifth *yama* that forbids greed, covetousness, and wastefulness

Asana (ā-): (1) physical posture (2) third limb of *Ashtanga Yoga*

Asat (a-saṭ; non-*sat*): false, unreal, non-existent

---

168 TRANSLITERATION KEY
a (org*a*n), **ā** (f*a*ther), **i** (p*i*n), **ī** (p*i*que), **u** (p*u*ll), **ū** (r*u*le), **ṛ** (fib*re*), **e** (th*ey*), and **o** (b*o*ne)
b, h, j, k, l, m, n, p, r, s, v, and **y** have usual English values; **g** as in *g*old;
j (*j*ug), **ch** (*ch*ur*ch*), and **ś** (*sh*ip) involve similar oral effort (*palatal*);
t, d, ṣ (sh), **ṇ** are uttered with retroflexed tongue (*lingual*);
ṭ, ṭh (*th*in), **ḍ** (*th*en), and **ḍh** (wi*thh*old) are *dental* sounds;
ḥ indicates aspiration; **ň, ñ, ṇ, n, m**, and **ṃ** indicate nasal sounds;
bh (jo*b h*ouse), **dh** (a*dh*ere), and so on.

Asatya (a-saṭya; non-*satya*): false, wrong, immoral, unreasonable, unjustifiable

Ashtanga Yoga (aṣṭāṅga-): Eight-limbed Yoga (not eight stepped or staged) comprising *yama, niyama, asana, pranayama, pratyahara, dharana, dhyana,* and *samadhi*

Asmita (-ṭā): (1) literally, am-ness (2) second *klesha* described as egoism (an erroneous and illusive identity) – however, with *viveka* it turns into *samadhi* of pure being!

Asteya (-ṭ-): (1) honesty, non-stealing (2) third *yama* that regards nothing worth stealing

Atma/Atman (āṭ-): noumenon, essential (core) Self [that is implicit in the term *Drashtri* (Seer/Knower)]; also called *Purusha*

Avagati (-ṭi): term used by philosopher *Shankara* for consciousness

Avidya (a-viḍyā): (1) ignorance of reality; non-*vidya* (2) primary and root *klesha* (Misery) (3) misjudging impermanent (aniṭya, or non-niṭya), impure (aśuchi, or non-śuchi), pain (*duhkha*), or non-self (anāṭma, or un-*atma*) as opposite

Aviveka: non-*viveka; samyoga;* knowledge contrary to *viveka*

Bhartrihari: 6th century AD philosopher poet [verses quoted are from his work on *vairagya*.]

Bhoga: (1) experience that deludes as real and meaningful (2) inability to distinguish between *Drashtri* (Self) and *drishya* (non-self) and consequent delusion of fulfilment from outside objects (3) upabhoga – the preposition upa emphasises quasi or illusory character of experience [q.v. *upalabdhi*]

Brahma/Brahman: the indivisible, all-encompassing Being; precisely, *Sat-Chit-Ananda*

Brahmacharya: fourth *yama* calling for broadmindedness and temperance

Chit/Chiti (ṭ): Consciousness (*Purusha*) or *Avagati*

Chitta (-ṭṭ-): mind – closest medium or accessory (anṭaḥ-karaṇa), but indeed an object of *Chiti*

Chitta-vritti (chiṭṭa-vṛṭṭi): any of five mental processes or modifications *viz.* right knowledge (*pramana*), illusion (*viparyaya*), fancy/delusion (*vikalpa*), sleep (*nidra*), and memory (*smriti*)

Darshana (ḍarśana): (1) literally, seeing (knowing) – it is commonly mistaken for philosophy and knowledgeable theories (which should technically be called *drishya*) (2) witnessing (3) vision

Dharana (ḍhāraṇā): sixth limb of *Ashtanga Yoga* called Concentration (attention held on a physical, here-now object/activity)

Dharma (ḍh-): (1) nature, law, quality, or characteristic (2) moral, righteous – as it ought to be (3) it is commonly mistaken for religion

Dhyana (ḍhyāna): seventh limb of *Ashtanga Yoga* called Contemplation (an uninterrupted session of *dharana*)

Drashtri (ḍraṣṭṛ): Seer/Knower or Consciousness [implicitly, Self]

drishya (ḍṛśya): (1) literally, worth-seeing or seeable – 'seeable' is a non-standard word, but aptly conveys core sense 'worth-knowing or knowable' (2) implicitly, it is non-self

Drishya (ḍṛśya): totality of all *drishyas*; Nature (*Prakriti*)

Duhkha (ḍuḥkha): pain – it arises from non-self

Dvesha (ḍveṣa): fourth *klesha* meaning hatred or aversion (targeted at sources of pain or discomfort) – pain (*duhkha*) provokes, or lies at the heart of, dvesha

Guna (-ṇa): (1) quality, attribute, humour, characteristic, or disposition (2) any of three fundamental constituents or attributes of Nature (*Prakriti*), namely: *sattva, rajas,* and *tamas*

Hana (hā-): (1) escape, especially escaping pain (*duhkha*) (2) *Kaivalya*

Hana-upaya (hāna-upāya): (1) means of escape with regard to pain (*duhkha*) (2) *viveka*

Hatha Yoga: *yoga* more focused on *asana, pranayama,* and other physical purificatory processes

Hetu (ṭ): cause, reason, justification

Heya: (1) worth escaping; to be escaped (2) prospective pain, or pain yet to come [In *Yoga* heya means both.]

Heya-hetu (ṭ): (1) literally, cause of pain (2) *samyoga*

Isha-vasya (īśā-vāsya): (1) literally, fit to be inhabited or pervaded by Lord [God] (2) principle of 'life divine'

Ishvara (īś-): (1) literally, lord, authority, ruler, almighty (2) God

Ishvara-pranidhana (-praṇiḍhāna): fifth *niyama* enjoining surrender to Lord Almighty

Kaivalya (kāi-): (1) aloneness but without plaintive yearning for company and possessions (2) establishment in Self (3) intrinsic (unarranged/effortless) liberation (4) name of fourth chapter of *Yoga* [q.v. *hana*]

Karma: (1) literally, action, work (2) past actions influencing one's current and future choices (actions) [q.v. *klesha-chain*]

Karma-chain: *klesha-chain*

Kartritva (karṭṛṭva): conceited sense of choice, agency (doership), and authority

Khyati (-āṭi): revelation, realisation, display

Klesha (kleśa): any of five Miseries (or causes of misery), namely: *Avidya*, egoism (*asmita*), pleasure-seated attachment (*raga*), pain-seated hatred/aversion (*dvesha*), and yearning for life (*abhinivesha*, or fear of death) [q.v. *klesha-chain*]

Klesha-chain: a self-feeding, ultimately-painful chain of *klesha*, *karma*, *phala*, and *samskara* [e.g., ignorance; wrongdoing; unwanted consequences; and inappropriate habits picked which again on finding suitable occasion and conditions restart the chain] — it manifests itself in train of births, life-spans, and painful experiences

Krishna (kṛṣṇa): Lord Krishna, eighth incarnation of Hindu God *Vishnu*

Lila (līlā): play, sport, diversion, amusement, pastime (unlike serious business)

Maya (māyā): (1) illusion (2) illusion-producing power

Mudra (-ḍrā): hand position, namely: Chin (*Chit*), *Vishnu*, Apana (-ā-), Shunya (śūnya), and Mrita Sanjivani (mṛṭa sañjīvanī) [chapter 2.4]

Narada (nāraḍa): bard of heavens and popular devotee of Lord *Vishnu*, mentioned in *The Puranas*

Neti neti (neṭi neṭi): admonition 'not this, not this' that signifies that Reality or Self is unknowable (or distinct from *Drishya*)

Nidra (-ḍrā): (1) dreamless (non-REM) sleep (2) fourth *chitta-vritti* (mental process) that is based on notional (not necessarily actual) 'non-existence' of objects

Nirodha (-ḍ-): practice and detachment (*vairagya*) with regard to mental processes (*chitta-vrittis*)

Niyama: second limb of *Ashtanga Yoga* comprising five rules, namely: *shaucha, santosha, tapas, svadhyaya,* and *Ishvara-pranidhana*

Om: (1) the most sacred and mystical syllable — figuratively represented by symbol ॐ (2) it is composed of three letters a, u, m (3) also called Pranava (ṇ) and *Omkar*

Omkar (oṅkāra; *om*-kāra): chant of *Om* (ॐ)

Parartha (parārṭha; para-arṭha meaning other-sake): (1) for the sake of or by virtue of another and not self (2) not self-existent (i.e., not existing absolutely, but relatively)

Parvati (pārvaṭī): wife of Hindu god *Shiva*

Patanjali (paṭañjali): Sage Patanjali who composed yoga sutras or *Yoga*

Phala: fruit, result, or consequence [q.v. *klesha-chain*]

Prajapati (prajāpaṭi): lord of creatures; creator [God]

Prakriti (-kṛṭi; Nature): elemental three *gunas* (efficient causes) together with their effect or modification (vikṛṭi) in the form of world

Pramana (-āṇa): first *chitta-vritti* (mental process) — the process of right knowledge involving direct perception (praṭyakṣa), inference (anumāna), and authorities (āgama)

Pranayama (prāṇāyāma): (1) literally, source or dimension of life (2) fourth limb of *Ashtanga Yoga* known as breathing exercises

Pratyahara (praṭyāhāra): fifth limb of *Ashtanga Yoga* involving withdrawal of senses from sense and thought objects

Purana (-āṇa): (1) any of a class of Hindu writings on myths and legends (2) Hindu mythology

Purusha (puruṣa): (1) Consciousness (*Chit/Chiti*) (2) essential Self (*Atman*) is the derived sense

Purusha-khyati: revelation or realisation (knowledge) of *Purusha* as essential Self (*Atman*)

Raga (rā-): third *klesha* meaning attachment [directed to sources of pleasure (*sukha*)] – love of pleasure lies at the heart of or generates raga

Raja Yoga (rā-): yoga of knowledge (it is suprerior and an end to *Hatha Yoga*)

Rajas: *guna* that signifies desire, passion, greed, sensuality, impulsion, action, motion, etc.

Sadhana (sāḍhana): (1) dedicated practice or learning (2) means (name of second chapter of *Yoga*)

Samadhi (-āḍhi): (1) *yoga* (2) eighth limb of *Ashtanga Yoga* signifying resolved state of mind – it is described as objective awareness and fictive personality [chapter 2.5] (3) name of first chapter of *Yoga*

Sambhuti (sambhūṭi): becoming, birth, or expansion

Samkalpa (ṃ): will, fancy, resolution – these are the ways mind operates

Samskara (saṃskāra): impression or tendency, having its root in memories of distant past [q.v. *klesha-chain*]

Samyak darshana: right vision (*viveka*)

Samyama (saṃ-): concurrence of *dharana, dhyana,* and *samadhi*

Samyoga (saṃ-; Conjunction): *aviveka;* obscurity about *viveka; heya-hetu*

Santosha (sanṭoṣa): second *niyama* signifying an attitude of contentment

Sat (-ṭ-): (1) real, existent, true (2) absolute reality or existence — one and only example is Consciousness [q.v. *asat*]

Sat-chit-ananda (alternatively, sachchiḍānanḍa): triune reality (*Brahma*) revealed as existence, consciousness, and bliss, respectively

Sattva (-ṭṭ-): *guna* that signifies essence, strength, illumination, knowledge, light, virtue, harmony, etc.

Satya (-ṭ-): (1) second *yama* enjoining truthfulness and integrity (2) literally, worth-existing or ideal (TRUTH IN PRINCIPLE) — it therefore stands for right, moral, reasonable, and righteous (3) living up to what one holds true; or conformity in thought, speech, and actions [q.v. *asatya*]

Savitri (-ṭṛ): Sun or creator god

Shankara (śaṅkara): (1) beneficent, auspicious (2) name of Hindu god (3) name of *advaita* philosopher (8th century AD)

Shaucha (śâucha): first *niyama* that calls for a favourable attitude to cleanliness, hygiene, and purity

Shiva (śiva): (1) auspicious, propitious, agreeable (2) a Hindu god

Shiva samkalpa: non-discriminatory good will

Smriti (smṛṭi): fifth *chitta-vritti* (mental process) meaning memory

Sukha: pleasure (which is transitory — subject to cause and effect) — like *duhkha*, it arises from non-self

Surya Namaskar (sūrya namaskāra): (1) literally, Sun Salutation (2) physical breath-synchronised movements through certain simple but vital *asanas*

Sutra (sūṭra): (1) literally, thread, string (2) threadlike proposition or definition; aphorism

Svadhyaya (svāḍhyāya = sva-aḍhyāya; self-study): fourth *niyama* involving study of scriptures conducted for enquiry into Self (*Atman*)

Svartha (svārṭha; sva-arṭha meaning self-sake): (1) for oneself; for one's own sake; or selfish (2) that exists by itself or for its own sake (self-existent, or existing absolutely)

Svayambhu (-ū): (1) self-existent [God] (2) Consciousness

Tamas (ṭ-): *guna* signifying ignorance, vice, delusion, darkness, inertia, dullness, passivity, heaviness, mass, etc.

Tapas (ṭ-): third *niyama* calling for forbearance and endurance toward difficulties faced in the path of yoga

Trishna (ṭṛṣṇā): greed, covetousness; *tamas-rajas* combo (ignorance in action)

Upalabdhi (-ḍhi): quasi (or façade of) gain or achievement; gainlike – term was used by philosopher *Shankara* for mental process or modification possibly to emphasise illusory character of life. Word is parallel to English word 'grasp' that means 'to seize' as well as 'to perceive, sense.' [q.v. *bhoga*]

Upanishad (-ṣaḍ): (1) esoteric doctrine (2) one of a series of post-*Veda* treatises on Vedic philosophy (especially monism) (3) source book of *Vedanta*

Upaya (-ā-): means, method [q.v. *hana-upaya*]

Vairagya (vāirāgya): detachment

Veda (ḍ): (1) knowledge (2) one of the four most ancient Hindu scriptures, namely: Rig (ṛg), Yajur, Sama (sā-), and Atharva (ṭ)

Vedanta (veḍānṭa; *veda*-anṭa): (1) end/conclusion/purport of knowledge or *The Veda* (2) Hindu monistic philosophy

Vibhuti (vibhūṭi): (1) glory (2) name of third chapter of *Yoga*

Vidya (-ḍyā): knowledge of reality

Vikalpa: third *chitta-vritti* (mental process) meaning fancy (delusion)

Viparyaya: second *chitta-vritti* (mental process) described as false or illusory impression of an actual stimulus/object

Vishnu (viṣṇu; all-pervader and mover): (1) Hindu God with incarnations as Rama (rā-), *Krishna*, and the Buddha (-ḍḍh-) (2) a *mudra*

Viveka: (1) *Drashtri-Drishya* distinction – Knower [Self] is different from known or knowable [non-self] (2) *hana-upaya*

Vivekin: one who is ever mindful of *viveka; yogin*

Vritti (vṛṭṭi): process [q.v. *chitta-vritti*]

Vyasa (-ā-): Sage Vyasa, the original (earliest) commentator of *Yoga*

Yajña: sacrifice (an act that is not primarily selfish and seeks to achieve welfare of all)

Yama: first limb of *Ashtanga Yoga* comprising mandatory but redeeming principles, namely: *ahimsa, satya, asteya, brahmacharya,* and *aparigraha*

yoga: (1) *samadhi* – not a union, unification, or achievement (2) *Kaivalya* (3) *Purusha-khyati* (4) yoga philosophy and discipline

Yoga: the book *Yoga Sutras* of *Patanjali*

Yogi (-ī; masculine)/**Yogini** (-ī; feminine)/**Yogin**: one with unceasing and unflinching commitment to *yoga* or *viveka*

APPENDIX B

Teacher-Disciple Dialogue

❄

EXCERPTS FROM
BOOK OF THOUSAND ADVICES
OF PHILOSOPHER SHANKARA

[Translation is close and not literal so that reader feels at home. Explanation where felt necessary is provided in square brackets. Original text appears in Appendix D.]

Disciple sums up: 'Sir, if this is so, [then conclusively] **Consciousness** (*avagati*) is self-evident, being verily self-intimating [known by itself] — in itself not requiring other evidence. [It exists absolutely, or is self-existent. Implicitly, it is **Self**. One can not deny one's existence.]

'All else is unconscious that combines and exists by virtue of or for the sake of another [Consciousness]. UNCONSCIOUS EXISTS AS WAYS OF THINKING and may not exist by itself or objectively in the same way! This explains quasi or paradoxical character of non-self objects that sometimes appear as pleasure, sometimes as pain, and sometimes as delusion. [They are therefore fit to be called *appearances*![169] Nothing other than Consciousness really exists!] Furthermore, as commonly experienced rope-snake, mirage-water, et al do not exist *except in our knowledge or mind*, then it is unreasonable to believe objects of waking and dream states as existing in reality (independent of our knowledge of them)!

'Sir, this self-luminous **Consciousness** is eternal and changeless by virtue of its subsistence throughout experience of

---

[169] They depend upon Consciousness for their manifestation.

objects. [Its denial is inconceivable! Without it nothing can be experienced!] Further, It alone exists as all else was seen above as appearances or as ways of thinking and also because objects of experience emerge and recede as phases.

'As in dreams the colourful variety of objects captures our attention [and deludes us] while it does not actually exist there, so in waking state object-variety likewise captures our attention and might not be actually existing! [That explains our oft subjective responses!]

'As It is known by Itself and none other, so It can not be accepted/secured or rejected/shed by Itself. Nothing else really exists!' [US II 109]

Teacher endorses and pinpoints the cause of pain: 'It is verily like that. It is Avidya[170] that projects transitory world (*saṃsāra*) composed of waking and dream experiences — deluding individuals as real and meaningful! Vidya [this much knowledge itself] wipes out Avidya. Thus you reclaim enduring fearlessness. You shall never suffer pain, whether awake or in dream; you are *indeed* delivered from worldly pain.' [US II 110]

Om! (ॐ) — thus hails the disciple. [US II 111] …

Non-self object is dubitable — this serves as ultimate argument. [US III 116]

One committed to ultimate vision therefore ought to give up all actions and their accessories like thread ceremony and others — all these being instigated by Avidya (ignorance). [US II 44]

[Had karma-chain been real, who could have escaped it!]

---

170 Refer to succinct yoga sutra on Avidya [II 5] or, for detail, section Avidya.

APPENDIX C

Yoga Sutras of Patanjali[171]

❋

SUTRAS IN ORIGINAL IN APPENDIX D

QUARTER I

Samadhi

1. Now is undertaken the authority/discipline of yoga for exposition.

2. *Yoga* is inhibition (nirodha) of mental processes (chitta-vrittis).

3. Then is the establishment of Seer Self (Drashtri) in essential/own nature.

4. Otherwise, there results conformity (identification) with mental processes.

5. Mental processes are of five types. These further are of two types – producing misery[172] and not producing misery.

6. These mental processes are right knowledge (pramana), illusion (viparyaya), fancy (vikalpa), sleep (nidra), and memory (smriti).

7. Process of *right knowledge* (*pramana*) involves direct perception, inference, and scriptural and other authorities.

8. *Illusion* (*viparyaya*) is false knowledge in the sense that perceived form or characteristic is not inherent in the object. [An *actual* object is misjudged here.]

---

[171] Instead of Sutras, word darshana is also used in some texts. It literally means knowing/seeing and not philosophy, knowledge, or certain dogmas. Yoga is witnessing (or Viveka in practice).

[172] Word used in original sutra is suggestive of Klesha (Misery) which is to be discussed in Quarter II.

9. *Fancy* (*vikalpa*) is image or concept of an object that looks probable but does not exist. [Object of fancy is *pseudo.*]

10. Mental process *sleep* (*nidra*) rests on the notion of non-existence of objects. [It is dreamless sleep, or NREM (non-rapid eye movement) phase of sleep.]

11. *Memory* (*smriti*) is reminding past experience of an object.

12. *Inhibition* (*nirodha*) of mental process is brought about by practice and detachment (vairagya).

13. *Practice* is effort for steadiness. [This effort is basically commitment.]

14. And practice maintained with dedication and uninterrupted in time gets firmly established.

15. Self-mastery in the sense of freedom from thirst or greed (Trishna) for perceived and heard-of[173] objects is called detachment (vairagya) of *subjugation* kind.

16. Next comes *superior* (or instinctive) *detachment* which is indeed guna-indifference[174] delivering one from worldly selfish concerns. This detachment comes from within — from knowledge of Purusha or Self (Purusha-khyati).

17. [With subjugation comes] *cognitive samadhi* which progresses through forms of speculation/vacillation, reflection/deliberation, exultation (ananda), and self-absorption (asmita, I-am-ness).

18. And with practised cessation of all desires (*i.e.*, superior detachment) [or with ceaseless inhibition of *all* mental processes] comes the other, *non-cognitive samadhi* in which impressions (samskaras) may remain [in order to carry on current life].

19. 'Bodiless Beings' and 'Beings Absorbed in Nature' classes of yogis realise this non-cognitive samadhi from birth by virtue of their having attained ananda and asmita samadhis, respectively, in their previous life.

20. For others practising inhibition now, this non-cognitive samadhi succeeds trust, perseverance, recollection (smriti), cognitive samadhi, and wisdom.

---

173 Such as mentioned in scriptures

174 For example, indifference to pleasure (*sattva*), pain (*rajas*), and delusion and inertia (*tamas*)

21. It is closer for those who ardently practise it.

22. A further three-fold distinction is there among those ardently practising: mild, moderate, and intense.

23. Alternatively, yoga (samadhi) is realised from surrender to Lord Almighty (Ishvara-pranidhana).

24. Lord (Ishvara) can be described as universal[175] Being or Consciousness (Purusha) untouched by either of Kleshas (Miseries), acts (karmas), fruits (consequences), and impressions (samskaras).

25. He is the ultimate seat or nucleus of omniscient intelligence. [He is the Knower (Seer, Consciousness) within all beings.]

26. With no gaps in time, He is guide (guru) of even the most ancient teachers.

27. He is expressed through sacred syllabic sound *Om* (ॐ). [Three constituent letters a, u, m of *Om* correspond to individual's roles or states as Waker, Dreamer, and Sleeper, respectively.]

28. To intone ॐ is to realise His essence as Self within [witness of, and distinct from, Drishya, phenomena, and roles].

29. This provides true and dispassionate perspective of life; establishes one in Self; and removes obstacles in the path of yoga.

30. Illness, sloth, indecision, carelessness, laziness, failure to withdraw (sensuality), delusional thinking, failure to attain Samadhi, and failure to retain Samadhi: these *mental projections* are the obstacles (distractions) in the path of yoga.

31. Pain (duhkha), rancour, physical restlessness, and irregular breathing accompany these projections.

32. To overcome these, practise one principle [like *Isha-vasya* (all as manifestation of one) and *fairness*].

33. Mind settles on cultivation of: friendliness toward joyful ones, instead of jealousy and envy; compassion toward suffering ones, instead of apathy and fault-finding; happiness at (or willing cooperation with) pious people, instead of deserting and purging them; and indifference (non-cooperation) toward impious people, instead of helping and approving their acts;

---

175 The adjective *viśeṣa* can be explained as 'nothing left out' (or excluding nothing).

34. Or [achieve the same] with breath [repeatedly] expelled and blocked out;

35. Or *attentive* physical or mental activity undertaken restores stability of mind;

36. So too, attention on the inner radiance [Consciousness!], which is free from sorrow[176];

37. So does company of (or attuning to) someone wise who mentally harbours no attachment [and greed] for objects and status or who has fulfilled purpose of life;

38. Likewise, if you include dream and sleep (nidra) in perspective [and correct your bias for waking life];

39. Or, lastly, achieve the same through Contemplation (dhyana) of whatever appealing or esteemed. [Contemplation is not limited to a few, countable ways!]

40. His mastery [what was called 'subjugation'] extends from objective (gross) atoms to subjective (subtle) individuality.

41. With mental processes[177] subdued, mind — like a flawless crystal absorbing whatever placed before it — assumes the form of that to which it is applied, whether cogniser, process of cognition, or object of cognition. Such conscious absorption [which was the subject matter of sutras 35-39 *supra*] is samadhi itself.

42. There, in *rough* speculation (vacillation) type, object of attention is crowded by notions of words, meanings, and intentions/theories. [It can also be translated as *with* speculation.]

43. [Next] comes *smooth* speculation (vacillation) with confusion of memory (smriti) abated. It is characterised as: (1) shining forth objects objectively, as they are; and (2) seemingly devoid or forgetful of own nature. [It can also be translated as *without* speculation. Here, knowledge becomes objective and humble (non-authoritative).[178]]

44. In the same fashion, reflection (deliberation) associated with subtle objects of attention can be explained as *rough* (or with) and *smooth* (or without).

---

[176] Pain and sorrow arise from non-self (duality).

[177] Not necessarily 'all' mental processes

[178] Refer to chapter 2.5 for detailed explanation.

45. Range of subtlety of objects extends to formless, elemental Nature (Prakriti).

46. These four are Samadhi but are *with seed* (*i.e.*, with pitfalls of Kleshas and Samskaras).

47. With refinement of the fourth Samadhi *smooth reflection* [*i.e.*, when even thought of no-thought has disappeared], Self reveals itself (or there is serenity within).

48. There, wisdom is replete with Truth [events are seen *as they are actually unfolding*].[179]

49. Unlike usual knowledge, this wisdom does not employ authority and inference obsessively. It is truly objective and comprehensive in quality.

50. Impression (samskara) born of it blocks further impressions (samskaras).

51. On inhibition of (or not yearning for) that (blissful) impression even — from inhibition (nirodha) of *all* — there emerges the [ultimate] *Seedless Samadhi* (*i.e.*, one free from potential Kleshas and Samskaras).

---

[179] A here-and-now interface

QUARTER II

Sadhana (Means)

1. Tapas (austerity, endurance), Svadhyaya (study of Self), and Ishvara-pranidhana (surrender to Lord Almighty): these three constitute *practical path to yoga* for …

2. … realisation of Samadhi and attenuation of Kleshas.

3. Avidya (Ignorance of Reality), Ego (asmita), Attachment (raga), Aversion or Hatred (dvesha), and Yearning for Life (abhinivesha) are the five *Miseries* (*Kleshas*).

4. Avidya acts as breeding ground for the latter four Miseries, whether they be dormant, attenuated, suspended, or operative (active).

5. *Avidya* (*Ignorance of Reality*) can be defined as perceiving or misjudging impermanent, impure, pain (duhkha), and non-self as permanent, pure, pleasure (sukha), and Self (Atma), respectively. [*Any* of these four misjudgements is Avidya.]

6. *Ego* (*asmita*) is assumed (iva) identity (oneness) between cogniser-faculty (Drashtri/Knower) and cognition-faculty (senses, mind, intellect, and also knowledge).

7. *Attachment* (*raga*) is rooted in or feeds on pleasure (sukha).

8. *Hatred* or *Aversion* (*dvesha*) is rooted in or feeds on pain (duhkha).

9. *Yearning for life*, or habitual fear of death (*abhinivesha*) feeds on itself and remains deep-seated in learned as well.

10. Those subtle Miseries are escaped with roll-back (or self-fulfilment).

11. Their processes are escaped with Contemplation called Dhyana [or with Viveka].

12. *Impressions of past good and bad actions* forming merit-demerit residuum or reservoir are rooted in Miseries (Kleshas). These impressions manifest (bear fruit) in current and unseen (future) lives.

13. As long as root [Kleshas — rather Avidya] is there, fruit is inevitable in the forms of births, life spans, and experiences

(bhogas) …

14. … which produce happiness and sorrow depending on excess of merit and demerit in balance, respectively.

15. For reasons of pain from change/transformation, anguish, and impressions (samskaras) and by virtue of conflicting guna-processes (guna-vrittis): all is indeed pain (duhkha) to vivekin (man of Viveka).

16. *Heya* (literally, to be escaped) stands for pain (duhkha) yet to come.

17. ***Samyoga*** (***Conjunction***) is lack of discrimination with regard to Drashtri (literally, seer/knower) and Drishya (literally, seeable/knowable). It is heya-hetu (cause of pain).

18. ***Drishya*** [***world***] is described as: (I) having the attributes (gunas) of *sattva* [which stands for light, knowledge], *rajas* [which stands for motion, desire, anger, greed, passion, activity], and *tamas* [which stands for mass, inertia, dullness, ignorance]; (II) assuming form of gross elements, senses, and ego (personality); and (III) providing experience (bhoga) to the ignorant and liberation (apavarga) to the enlightened.

19. Gunas evolve in four steps: sixteen *particulars*[180], six *non-particulars*[181], *mere form* (*Great Principle*[182]); and formless Prakriti (Nature).

20. *Drashtri* (*Seer*) is just seeing/knowing (consciousness) which even though pure resembles or is identified with objects like thoughts etc. [Fall from purity is the result of oversight of Viveka!]

21. Drishya exists verily for the sake of or by virtue of Drashtri.[183]

22. Drishya (world) disappears for the enlightened one[184], but it

---

[180] Five gross elements (ether, air, fire, water, earth), five corresponding sense organs (ear, skin, eye, tongue, nose), five organs of action (hands, feet, larynx, organs of reproduction and excretion), and mind

[181] Ego-sense and five subtle elements (sound, touch, form, taste, smell)

[182] Intelligence (mahaṭ) [but not Witness (sākṣin)/Purusha/Drashtri]

[183] It is analogous to beauty! As beauty is *relative* (it lies in the eye of the beholder), so too, Drishya (world) – it appears differently to different people. For some, it disappears too as said in the next sutra.

commonly exists for others. [Others have not realised it as *appearance* so far!]

23. Samyoga serves to reveal distinction between possessor and possessed (or Self and non-self).

24. Avidya is the cause (hetu) of this Samyoga (Drashtri-Drishya Conjunction).

25. As Avidya ceases, so does Samyoga; this is *Escape* (hana), or *Liberation* (***Kaivalya***[185]) of Drashtri from the painful world.

26. Unbroken display/practice of **Viveka** (Drashtri-Drishya Distinction[186]) is the *means of escape* (*hana-upaya*).

27. Wisdom of Vivekin is ultimate, seven-typed.

28. On destruction of impurities with observance of yoga limbs, knowledge climaxes in Viveka.

29. Yama, niyama, asana, pranayama, pratyahara, dharana, dhyana, and samadhi: these eight limbs form *Ashtanga Yoga.* [Caution: it is not eight-staged.]

30. Ahimsa (non-violence), satya (truthfulness, integrity), asteya (non-stealing, honesty), brahmacharya (broadminded, devout life), and aparigraha (non-covetousness) form the first limb. They are called *yamas* (or laws of life).

31. Yamas are mandatory — to be observed by all regardless of time, place, birth/caste, or eventuality. They form a solemn vow.

32. Shaucha (purity), santosha (contentment), tapas (austerity, endurance), svadhyaya (study of scriptures aimed at knowledge of Self), and Ishvara-pranidhana (surrender to Lord Almighty): they are *niyamas* (or personal rules), the second limb.

33. When challenged by negative (tempting) arguments, reflect over the opposite.

34. Violence etc. – whether done, caused, or condoned and

---

[184] One who has realised purpose of life or who has no purpose of life to be fulfilled

[185] It is the state of aloneness without the plaintive yearning for company and possessions.

[186] This is also called Mind-Purusha Distinction (Sattva-Purusha Distinction) that stresses that mind in its pure form (*sattva*) is still Prakriti and distinct from Purusha.

whether mild, moderate, or intense – are incited by greed, anger, and delusion. They result in endless ignorance and pain (duhkha). Thus is reflected the opposite.

35. On establishment in ahimsa, life around devotee becomes hostility-free.

36. Establishment in satya makes actions bear fruits.

37. With establishment in asteya, riches of world (literally, all jewels) converge at him.

38. With establishment in brahmacharya comes increase in potency.

39. With steadiness in aparigraha comes insight into purpose (wherefore) of life/birth.

40. From shaucha arises disenchantment with one's own body and contact with others (*e.g.*, coitus) …

41. and also come along: mental (intentional) purity, beneficence, one-pointedness, mastery of senses, and fitness for self-realisation (Atma-darshana).

42. From santosha is gained unparalleled happiness (sukha).

43. On elimination of impurities from tapas comes perfection of body and senses.

44. Svadhyaya brings communion with personal, favourite deity. [It rather implants cherished values and virtues!]

45. From Ishvara-pranidhana comes perfection of samadhi.

46. The third limb, *asana* (physical posture) affords steadiness and repose (sukha) …

47. … through relaxation of effort and absorption in the Infinite, Absolute [Brahma].

48. Thence, dualities of life such as pleasure-pain and hot-cold do not disturb the yoga devotee (not simply asana fan).

49. Asana-onward [with mind and body settled], there arises the fourth limb, *pranayama* (life-expansive energy; or higher dimension/source of life energy) associated with natural suspension of flow of breath. [Rapid and shallow breathing is an indicator of disturbed mood and emotions!]

50. Pranayama can be distinguished in terms of location, duration, and number; and inhaling, exhaling, and stalling (retention of breath) can be proactively regulated in order to make it deep and subtle.

51. Sphere of the fourth Pranayama lies beyond incoming and outgoing breaths. [It is the natural Pranayama of sutra 49.]

52. Thence veil of light gets destroyed.

53. Besides, there arises fitness of mind for dharana (concentration), the sixth yoga limb.

54. When senses no longer savour objects, they assume the form of mind. This is *pratyahara* (withdrawal of senses), the fifth limb of yoga.

55. Thence arises absolute mastery of senses.

QUARTER III

Vibhuti (Glory)

[*Powers elude power-seekers! They naturally rush in resolved minds!*]

1. Attention held on a definite locus [physical, here-now object/activity] is *dharana* (concentration), the sixth limb of yoga. [Objects far-away in space or time can turn fanciful and therefore distractive!]

2. When object of attention there [in dharana] is uniform, it is *dhyana* (contemplation), the seventh limb. [It is a longer session of dharana on a single object/activity.]

3. Further, when object of attention shines forth as it is [objectively] and in a self-forgetful state (as if devoid of own nature)[187] — it is *samadhi (meditation)*, the eighth limb of yoga.

4. When the three: dharana, dhyana, and samadhi are concurrent, it is *samyama.*

5. From perfection (command) in it, wisdom dawns.

6. It should be applied in various states of chitta.

7. Last three limbs are internal in relation to the former, five limbs.

8. However, they [three limbs] are external in relation to Seedless Samadhi.

9. *Nirodha transformation of mind* happens the moment impression (samskara) of extroversion is overpowered by emerging impression (samskara) of nirodha (inhibition, detachment).

10. Its tranquil flow is by reasons of the nirodha samskara.

11. *Samadhi transformation of mind* is the disappearance of all-pointedness (or dispersiveness) and rise of one-pointedness in mind.

---

[187] Knowing is one's nature and not knowledge that keeps changing. So there can be no claim for knowledge here (or seemingly not knowing). Here knowledge becomes objective and humble (non-authoritative – free from dogma and self-conceit).

12. Thereafter comes *one-pointed transformation of mind* in which subsiding and rising objects remain similar.

13. Likewise are described transformations of characteristic (dharma), time-phase, and state seen in the gross elements and senses.

14. The object in which reside quiescent [no more active], active, and impending (yet to be active) characteristics (dharmas) is called *object characterised*[188].

15. Different sequence produces difference in transformations.

16. From samyama on three transformations comes knowledge of past and future.

17. Words, meanings, and purports overlap and delude. However, from samyama on their distinctiveness comes understanding of sounds of all beings or creatures.

18. From samyama on samskaras (impressions) comes knowledge of previous lives/births.

19. From samyama on someone's thought comes knowledge of other's mind or intention.

20. However object of intention of the other can not be known; that can not be object of samyama.

21. From samyama on the form of body is hampered perceptibility of body, with contact between eye and light severed. Thus is achieved imperceptibility of body.

22. Karma fruition is fast or slow. From samyama on it or from portents is gained foreknowledge of death.

23. From samyama on friendliness etc. [mentioned in I 33] arises fortitude.

24. Samyama on strengths produces strengths *viz.* of elephant.

25. From direction of light of inner radiance [mentioned in I 36] can be gained clairvoyance of subtle, hidden, and remote objects.

26. Knowledge of worlds or Solar System comes from samyama on the Sun.

27. From samyama on the Moon comes knowledge of

---

[188] ḍharmī or ḍharmin

constellations (or arrays of stars).

28. From samyama on the Pole Star comes knowledge of their motions with reference to it.

29. From samyama on navel plexus (also called solar plexus) comes knowledge of bodily systems.

30. From samyama on throat cavity comes cessation of hunger and thirst.

31. From samyama on tortoise tube [below the throat cavity] is gained steadiness.

32. From samyama on the light in head, realised ones reveal themselves.

33. Alternatively, from intuitive perception [born of Samadhi], everything can be known.

34. From samyama on the heart (essential Self!) are comprehended mind and its processes.

35. *Bhoga*[189] (experience; enjoyment of objects) arises from oversight of distinction of sattva[190] and Purusha (Drashtri, Self) and exists for the sake of another. It is Parartha (relative). [That is why bhoga is regarded differently by different people!] Whereas Purusha is revealed from samyama on *'what exists for its own sake or by itself'* (Svartha; absolute existence or truth).

36. From that revelation of Purusha, intuitive hearing, touch, vision, taste, and smell arise.

37. They are indeed obstacles in samadhi, but are seen as perfections (powers) by extroverts. [Or they are bye-products of Samadhi and should not be aspired as separate ideals!]

38. From loosened karmic bond and from awareness of movements of mind is enabled entry of mind in others' bodies.

39. Triumph of *udana* (the air circulating in head) produces non-contact with water, mud, thorns, etc. and ascension to heavens at the time of death.

---

[189] It is no different from Samyoga. It is an illusory identification.

[190] It means mind, intellect, knowledge, righteousness, or essence. See explanation for Sattva-Purusha Distinction in the footnote of yoga sutra II 26.

40. Triumph of *samana* (the air distributing food equally to body) produces glow or halo.

41. Samyama on the relation between hearing and space produces supernatural hearing.

42. From samyama on the relation between body and space and from mental absorption on the lightness of cotton comes ability to traverse through space.

43. *The Great Without-Body* is the mental process that operates outside body and without imagination. Samyama on that destroys veil of light.

44. Samyama on gross forms, characteristics, essences, relationship, and purpose brings triumph of gross elements.

45. Thence arise (1) eight attainments such as attenuation etc., (2) elegance of body, and (3) non-obstruction by the characteristics of gross elements [*e.g.*, fire does not burn].

46. Beauty, grace, strength, and adamantine hardness — these constitute bodily elegance.

47. From samyama on power of perception, essential nature, I-am-ness (asmita), relationship, and purpose comes triumph of senses.

48. Therefrom emerge (1) swiftness as of mind, (2) operation independent of physical organs, and (3) conquest of Nature.

49. One who has realised distinctness of sattva[191] and Purusha only enjoys omnipotence and omniscience.

50. From detachment even toward that [Viveka], seed of evil [Kleshas] is destroyed — thus arises Kaivalya.

51. Fearing re-emergence of evil, one should not take interest or pride in alluring invitations of celestial deities (or influential beings).

52. From samyama on moments and their succession[192] comes knowledge born of Discrimination (Viveka).

---

[191] See footnotes of yoga sutras II 26 and III 35.

[192] Two moments can not coincide. One of the two has to be either antecedent or subsequent. Either way, one moment becomes non-existent. Concept of time as past and future is fanciful, hypothetical. Moreover, no event is purely past, future, or present. Same event can be past for one and future for other.

53. Thereby can be distinguished two things (in time), when they are otherwise similar in class (genus), characteristics, or location.

54. That discriminative knowledge is: intuitive or clairvoyant; knowing all objects and in all states; and unlike usual, progressive knowledge [that grows in volume over time and is not complete at any time].

55. (Even otherwise or anyway) when sattva and Purusha are cognised with equal clarity, there is *Kaivalya* (Enlightenment, or Liberation).

QUARTER IV

Kaivalya

1. Perfections (powers) result by virtue of birth, drugs, incantations, austerity (tapas), and samadhi.

2. Transformation into another life-state results from overflow of natural causes (Prakriti). [Purusha (Self) is not an agent of changes.]

3. Incidental causes do not change the nature (prakriti) of things or set things into action/motion, but only remove their obstacles, like a farmer does not irrigate by carrying water to fields but by removing barriers in the way of water. [Powers remove obstacles and do not produce samadhi. Open the door and let the sunshine in!]

4. Five created minds arise from ego (asmita) only.

5. One mind directs many created minds into various activities.

6. Among five perfected minds, mind born of dhyana (or samadhi) is free from impressions. [This mind is taintless.]

7. Karma of Yogi is neither pure (white) nor impure (black); but others' are three-fold (*i.e.*, pure, impure, and mixed).

8. Compatible with fruits of three-fold karma arise desires or aspirations (or fond memories).

9. Memories (smritis) and impressions (samskaras) being basically similar lurk around despite interruptions by birth, place, and time.

10. They are beginningless as self-interest is ever present.

11. Held together by cause (hetu), effect (phala), substratum (mind), and object, they (impressions) cease as these four cease.

12. Past and future indeed exist within an object as different ways or forms of characteristics (dharmas) operating at a certain time [as some having operated and some yet to operate].

13. These characteristics are manifest or subtle and embody the attributes (gunas).

14. From uniqueness of transformation emerges entity of an object.

15. Same object assumes different ways or forms due to difference in minds. [Things exist more as ways of thinking.]

16. But, if thing is postulated as a mental-construct alone, then what would happen to it when that object is not perceived! [Object should have physically disappeared! But that is not the case. This sutra should be read with yoga sutra II 22.]

17. Object is known or unknown depending on mind being coloured by it or not. [For us things exist when known and do not when not known! Yoga benefits one who knows yoga, and not others.]

18. Mental processes (chitta-vrittis) are always known to its (mind's) lord (prabhu) Purusha — latter being changeless.

19. It (mind) is not self-intimating, being knowable (drishya).

20. Two (mind and object) can not be cognised simultaneously.

21. Mind can be an object (drishya) of another subtler mind! — if this is postulated, this results in endless regress of cognisors and cognitions; and consequent confusion of memories.

22. Idea of self in mind is obtained when mind assumes that form of Consciousness (Chiti) which is unchanging (not moving from object to object). [This is obtained in a steady mind.]

23. Mind coloured by Seer (Drashtri) and seeable (drishya) is multipurpose. [For laypersons, mind is self and knower of objects. On the other hand, yogi knows mind as object of and different from Self. Simply said, yogi watches his mind and thus distinguishes Self from mind.[193]]

24. Though variegated by innumerable impressions, mind is not independent or competent by itself. It exists for the sake of another. [It is Parartha.]

25. For one who has realised the distinction comprehensively (or exclusively), there is cessation of cogitation or actualisation of Self (Atman).[194]

26. Then, viveka-inclined mind accelerates toward Kaivalya.

---

193 Consciousness is the perception of what passes in a man's own mind. (John Locke)

194 The word *bhāva* has two meanings: existence/state/entity and feeling/reflection.

27. In their intervals appear other thoughts due to impressions (samskaras).

28. Escape (hana) from them is similar to that stated for Miseries (Kleshas).

29. One disinterested even in the Highest Knowledge and scrupulously practising Viveka realises Bounty-of-Virtue Samadhi.

30. Thence arises cessation of Miseries (Kleshas) and activities (karma).

31. Then, freed from all impurities, knowledge becomes infinite and there is hardly anything left to be known.

32. Thence comes cessation of transformation process (*krama*, or succession) of attributes (gunas), having fulfilled their purpose.

33. *Succession* (*krama*) can be defined as: that is recognised as transformation stages concurrent with time (moments).

34. Attributes (gunas) when left with no purpose of Purusha to be served roll back (or dissolve). This is *Kaivalya,* described as establishment in Self (own nature). This is also called Power of Consciousness (Chiti[195]). *Finis.*

---

[195] It does not change. It does not move from object to object; rather objects are shown to It. It is pure and infinite. [Sage Vyasa's comments on yoga sutra I 2]

APPENDIX D

Sources in Sanskrit

❄

TRANSLITERATION KEY

<u>*Vowels*</u>: अ/**a** (org*a*n), आ/**ā** (f*a*ther), इ/**i** (p*i*n), ई/**ī** (p*i*que), उ/**u** (p*u*ll), ऊ/**ū** (r*u*le), ऋ/**ṛ** (fib*re*),

ए/**e** (th*ey*), ओ/**o** (b*o*ne), ऐ/**āi** (n*igh*t), औ/**āu** (h*ou*se)

<u>*Pure consonants*</u>: ब/**b**, ह/**h**, ज/**j**, क/**k**, ल/**l**, म/**m**, न/**n**, प/**p**, र/**r**, स/**s**, व/**v**, and य/**y** have usual English values; ग/**g** as in *g*old;

ज/**j** (*j*ug), च/**ch** (*ch*ur*ch*), and श/**ś** (*sh*ip) involve similar oral effort (*palatal*);

ट/**t**, ड/**d**, ष/**ṣ** (sh), ण/**ṇ** are uttered with retroflexed tongue (*lingual*);

त/**ṭ**, थ/**ṭh** (*th*in), द/**ḍ** (*th*en), and ध/**ḍh** (wi*thh*old) are *dental* sounds;

:/**ḥ** indicates aspiration; ङ/**ň**, ञ/**ñ**, **ṇ**, **n**, ˙/**m**, and ˘/**ṃ** indicate nasal sounds;

भ/**bh** (jo*b h*ouse), ढ/**dh** (a*dh*ere), ख/**kh** (ba*ck h*ome), घ/**gh** (*gh*ost), छ/**chh** (ba*tch h*ouse), झ/**jh** (ba*dge h*older), ठ/**th** (res*t h*ome), and फ/**ph** (u*ph*ill)

CHAPTER 3.1

ॐ My Mind be of Shiva Samkalpa! ॐ

यज्जाग्रतो दूरमुदैति दैवं तदु सुप्तस्य तथैवैति।

दूरङ्गमं ज्योतिषाञ्ज्योतिरेकं तन्मे मनः शिवसङ्कल्पमस्तु॥ [1]

येन कर्माण्यपसो मनीषिणो यज्ञे कृण्वन्ति विदथेषु धीराः।

यदपूर्वं यक्षमन्तः प्रजानां तन्मे मनः शिवसङ्कल्पमस्तु॥ [2]

यत्प्रज्ञानमुत चेतो धृतिश्च यज्ज्योतिरन्तरमृतं प्रजासु।

यस्मान्न ऋते किञ्चन कर्म क्रियते तन्मे मनः शिवसङ्कल्पमस्तु॥ [3]

येनेदं भूतं भुवनं भविष्यत्परिगृहीतममृतेन सर्वम्।

येन यज्ञस्तायते सप्तहोता तन्मे मनः शिवसङ्कल्पमस्तु॥ [4]

यस्मिन्नृचःसामयजूँषि यस्मिन्प्रतिष्ठिता रथनाभाविवाराः।

यस्मिंश्चित्तँ सर्वमोतं प्रजानां तन्मे मनः शिवसङ्कल्पमस्तु॥ [5]

सुषारथिरश्वानिव यन्मनुष्यान्नेनीयते अभीशुभिर्वाजिन इव।

हृत्प्रतिष्ठं यदजिरं जविष्ठं तन्मे मनः शिवसङ्कल्पमस्तु॥ [6]

yajjāgraṭo ḍūramuḍāiṭi ḍāivam ṭaḍu supṭasya ṭaṭhāivāiṭi; ḍūraṅgamam jyoṭiṣāñ jyoṭirekam ṭan me manaḥ śivasaṅkalpam aṣṭu. [1] yena karmānyapaso manīṣiṇo yajñe kṛṇvanṭi viḍaṭheṣu ḍhīrāḥ; yaḍapūrvam yakṣamanṭaḥ prajānām ... (Refrain) [2] yaṭ prajñānamuṭa cheṭo ḍhṛṭiścha yajjyoṭir anṭar amṛṭam prajāsu; yasmānna ṛṭe kiñchana karma kriyaṭe ... (Refrain) [3] yeneḍam bhūṭam bhuvanam bhaviṣyaṭ parigṛhīṭam amṛṭena sarvam; yena yajñasṭāyaṭe sapṭahoṭā ... (Refrain) [4] yasminnṛchaḥsāmayajūṃsi yasmin praṭiṣṭhiṭā raṭhanābhāvivārāḥ; yasmiñśchiṭṭam sarvamoṭam prajānām ... (Refrain) [5] suṣāraṭhiraśvāniva yan manuṣyānnenīyaṭe abhīśubhir vājina iva; hṛṭpraṭiṣṭham yaḍajiram javiṣṭham ... (Refrain) [6] (YV xxxiv 1-6)

CHAPTER 4.2

In Surrender to Him, Enjoy!

ईशा वास्यमिदँ सर्वं यत्किञ्च जगत्याञ्जगत्।

तेन त्यक्तेन भुञ्जीथा मा गृधः कस्यस्विद्धनम्॥ [1]

कुर्वन्नेवेह कर्माणि जिजीविषेच्छतँ समाः।

एवं त्वयि नान्यथेतोऽस्ति न कर्म लिप्यते नरे॥ [2]

īśā vāsyam iḍaṃ sarvam yaṭ kiñcha jagaṭyāñ jagaṭ; ṭena ṭyakṭena bhuñjīṭhā mā gṛḍhaḥ kasyasviḍḍhanam. [1] kurvanneveha karmāṇi jijīviṣechchhaṭaṃ samāḥ; evam ṭvayi nānyaṭheṭo'sṭi na karma lipyaṭe nare. [2] (IU 1-2)

CHAPTER 4.3

Prayer

ॐ विश्वानि देव सवितर्दुरितानि परा सुव। यद्भद्रं तन्न आ सुव॥ [1]

सर्वे भवन्तु सुखिनः सर्वे सन्तु निरामयाः।

सर्वे भद्राणि पश्यन्तु मा कश्चिद्दुःखभाग्भवेत्॥ [2]

प्रजापते न त्वदेतान्यन्यो विश्वा जातानि [रूपाणि] परि ता बभूव।

यत्कामास्ते जुहुमस्तन्नो अस्तु वयं स्याम पतयो रयीणाम्॥ [3]

असतो मा सद्गमय तमसो मा ज्योतिर्गमय मृत्योर्मामृतं गमय। [4]

om viśvāni ḍeva saviṭar ḍuriṭāni parā suva; yaḍ bhaḍram ṭanna ā suva. [1] (YV xxx 3)

sarve bhavanṭu sukhinaḥ sarve sanṭu nirāmayāḥ; sarve bhaḍrāṇi paśyanṭu mā kaśchiḍḍuḥkhabhāg bhaveṭ. [2]

prajāpaṭe na ṭvaḍeṭānyanyo viśvā jāṭāni [rūpāṇi] pariṭā babhūva; yaṭ kāmās ṭe juhumas ṭanno asṭu vayaṃ syāma paṭayo rayīṇām. [3] (RV X cxxi 10)

asaṭo mā saḍgamaya ṭamaso mā jyoṭirgamaya mṛṭyor māmṛṭam gamaya. [4] (BU I iii 28)

ॐ भूर्भुवः स्वः। तत्सवितुर्वरेण्यं भर्गो देवस्य धीमहि।

धियो यो नः प्रचोदयात्॥ [1]

भद्रं कर्णेभिः शृणुयाम देवा भद्रं पश्येमाक्षभिर्यजत्राः।

स्थिरैरङ्गैस्तुष्टुवाँसस्तनूभिर्व्यशेमहि देवहितं यदायुः॥ [2]

तच्चक्षुर्देवहितं पुरस्ताच्छुक्रमुच्चरत्।

पश्येम शरदः शतं जीवेम शरदः शतँ शृणुयाम शरदः शतं प्रब्रवाम

शरदः शतमदीनाः स्याम शरदः शतं भूयश्च शरदः शतात्॥ [3]

नमः शम्भवाय च मयोभवाय च नमः शङ्कराय च मयस्कराय च

नमः शिवाय च शिवतराय च॥ [4]

त्र्यम्बकं यजामहे सुगन्धिं पुष्टिवर्धनम्।

उर्वारुकमिव बन्धनान्मृत्योर्मुक्षीय मामृतात् ॥ [5]

अग्ने नय सुपथा राये अस्मान् विश्वानि देव वयुनानि विद्वान्।

युयोध्यस्मज्जुहुराणमेनो भूयिष्ठां ते नम उक्तिं विधेम॥ [6][196]

CHAPTER 4.4

God and My Identity

स पर्यगाच्छुक्रमकायमव्रणमस्नाविरँ शुद्धमपापविद्धम्।

कविर्मनीषी परिभूः स्वयम्भूर्याथातथ्यतोऽर्थान्व्यदधाच्छाश्वतीभ्यः समाभ्यः॥

sa paryagāchchhukram akāyam avraṇam asnāviraṃ śuḍḍham apāpaviḍḍham. kavir manīṣī paribhūḥ svayam-bhūr yāṭhāṭaṭhyaṭo'rṭhān vyaḍaḍhāchchhāśvaṭībhyaḥ samābhyaḥ. [IU 8]

---

[196] Om bhūr bhuvaḥ svaḥ. ṭaṭ saviṭur vareṇyam bhargo ḍevasya ḍhīmahi; ḍhiyo yo naḥ prachoḍayāṭ. [1] (YV xxxvi 3) bhaḍram karṇebhiḥ śṛṇuyāma ḍevā bhaḍram paśyemākṣabhir yajaṭrāḥ; sṭhirāiraṅgāis ṭuṣṭuvāṃsas ṭanūbhir vyaśemahi ḍevahiṭam yaḍāyuḥ. [2] (YV xxv 21) ṭachchakṣur ḍevahiṭam purasṭāchchhukram uchcharaṭ. paśyema śaraḍaḥ śaṭam jīvema śaraḍaḥ śaṭaṃ śṛṇuyāma śaraḍaḥ śaṭam prabravāma śaraḍaḥ śaṭamaḍīnāḥ syāma śaraḍaḥ śaṭam bhūyaścha śaraḍaḥ śaṭāṭ. [3] (YV xxxvi 24) namaḥ śambhavāya cha mayobhavāya cha namaḥ śaṅkarāya cha mayaskarāya cha namaḥ śivāya cha śivaṭarāya cha. [4] (YV xvi 41) ṭryambakam yajāmahe suganḍhim puṣṭivarḍhanam; urvārukam iva banḍhanān mṛṭyor mukṣīya māmṛṭāṭ. [5] (YV iii 60) agne naya supaṭhā rāye asmān viśvāni ḍeva vayunāni viḍvān; yuyoḍhyasmaj juhurāṇameno bhūyiṣṭhān ṭe nama ukṭim viḍhema. [6] (IU 18)

CHAPTER 6.4

I am Brahma

ब्रह्म वा इदमग्र आसीत्, तदात्मानमेवावेत्। अहं ब्रह्मास्मीति। तस्मात्तत्सर्वमभवत्। तद्यो यो देवानां प्रत्यबुध्यत, स एव तदभवत्। तथर्षीणां, तथा मनुष्याणाम्। तद्धैतत्पश्यन्नृषिर्वामदेवः प्रतिपेदे, अहं मनुरभवं सूर्यश्चेति। तदिदमप्येतर्हि य एवं वेद, अहं ब्रह्मास्मीति, स इदं सर्वं भवति, तस्य ह न देवाश्चना भूत्या ईशते। आत्मा ह्येषां स भवति; अथ योऽन्यां देवतामुपास्ते, अन्योऽसावन्योऽहमस्मीति, न स वेद, यथा पशुरेवं स देवानाम्।

brahma vā iḍam agra āsīṭ, ṭaḍāṭmānamevāveṭ. aham brahmāsmīṭi. ṭasmāṭṭaṭsarvam abhavaṭ. ṭaḍ yo yo ḍevānām praṭyabuḍhyaṭa, sa eva ṭadabhavaṭ. ṭaṭharṣīṇām, ṭaṭhā manuṣyāṇām. ṭaḍḍhāiṭaṭ paśyannṛṣir vāmaḍevaḥ praṭipeḍe, aham manurabhavam sūryaścheṭi. ṭaḍiḍam apyeṭarhi ya evam veḍa, aham brahmāsmīṭi, sa iḍam sarvam bhavaṭi, ṭasya ha na ḍevāśchanā bhūṭyā īśaṭe. āṭmā hyeṣām sa bhavaṭi; aṭha yo'nyām ḍevaṭāmupāsṭe, anyo'sāvanyo'ham asmīṭi, na sa veḍa, yaṭhā paśurevam sa ḍevānām. (BU I iv 10)

APPENDIX B

Teacher-Disciple Dialogue

यद्येवं भगवन् कूटस्थनित्यावगतिः आत्मज्योतिःस्वरूपैव स्वयंसिद्धा, आत्मनि प्रमाणनिरपेक्षत्वात्, ततोऽन्यत् अचेतनं संहत्यकारित्वात् परार्थम् । येन च सुखदुःखमोहप्रत्ययावगतिरूपेण पारार्थ्यं, तेनैव स्वरूपेण अनात्मनः अस्तित्वं, नान्येन रूपान्तरेण, अतो नास्तित्वमेव परमार्थतः। यथा हि लोके रज्जुसर्पमरीच्युदकादीनां तदवगतिव्यतिरेकेण अभावो दृष्टः, एवं जाग्रत्स्वप्न-द्वैतभावस्यापि तदवगतिव्यतिरेकेण अभावो युक्तः। एवमेव परमार्थतः भगवन् अवगतेः आत्मज्योतिषः नैरन्तर्यभावात् कूटस्थनित्यता, अद्वैतभावश्च, सर्वप्रत्ययभेदेषु अव्यभिचारात्। प्रत्ययभेदास्तु अवगतिं व्यभिचरन्ति। यथा स्वप्ने नीलपीताद्याकारभेदरूपाः प्रत्ययाः तदवगतिं व्यभिचरन्तः परमार्थतो न

सन्तीत्युच्यन्ते, एवं जाग्रत्यपि नीलपीतादिप्रत्ययभेदाः तामेवावगतिं व्यभिचरन्तः असत्यरूपा भवितुमर्हन्ति। तस्याश्चावगतेः अन्यः अवगन्ता नास्तीति न स्वेन स्वरूपेण स्वयं उपादातुं हातुं वा शक्यते, अन्यस्य च अभावात्॥[197]

तथैवेति। एषा अविद्या यन्निमित्तः संसारो जाग्रत्स्वप्नलक्षणः। तस्या अविद्यायाः विद्या निवर्तिका। इत्येवं त्वं अभयं प्राप्नोषि। नातः परं जाग्रत्स्वप्नदुःखमनुभविष्यसि, संसारदुःखान्मुक्तोऽसीति॥[198]

ओमिति॥[199] [US II 109-11]

अनात्मवस्तुनश्चासत्त्वात् इति परमो हेतुः।[200] [US III 116]

तस्मादविद्याकार्यत्वात् सर्वकर्मणां तत्साधनानां च यज्ञोपवीतादीनां

---

197 yaḍyevam bhagavan kūtasṭhanitṭyāvagaṭiḥ āṭmajyoṭiḥ svarūpāiva svayaṃsiḍḍhā, āṭmani pramāṇanirapekṣaṭvāṭ, ṭaṭo'nyaṭ acheṭanam saṃhaṭyakāriṭvāṭ parārṭham. yena cha sukhaḍuḥkhamoha-praṭyayāvagaṭirūpeṇa pārārṭhyam ṭenāiva svarūpeṇa anāṭmanaḥ asṭiṭvam nānyena rūpānṭareṇa, aṭo nāsṭiṭvameva paramārṭhaṭaḥ. yaṭhā hi loke rajjusarpamarīchyuḍakāḍīnām ṭaḍavagaṭivyaṭirekeṇa abhāvo ḍṛṣṭaḥ, evam jāgraṭsvapnaḍvāiṭabhāvasyāpi ṭaḍavagaṭivyaṭirekeṇa abhāvo yukṭaḥ. evameva paramārṭhaṭaḥ bhagavan avagaṭeḥ āṭmajyoṭiṣaḥ nāiranṭaryabhāvāṭ kūtasṭhaniṭyaṭā, aḍvāiṭabhāvaścha, sarvapraṭyayabheḍeṣu avyabhichārāṭ. praṭyayabheḍāsṭu avagaṭim vyabhicharanṭi. yaṭhā svapne nīlapīṭāḍyākārabheḍarūpāḥ praṭyayāḥ ṭaḍavagaṭim vyabhicharanṭaḥ paramārṭhaṭo na sanṭīṭyuchyanṭe, evam jāgraṭyapi nīlapīṭāḍipraṭyayabheḍāḥ ṭāmevāvagaṭim vyabhicharanṭaḥ asaṭyarūpā bhaviṭumarhanṭi. ṭasyāśchāvagaṭeḥ anyaḥ avaganṭā nāsṭīṭi na svena svarūpeṇa svayam upāḍāṭum hāṭum vā śakyaṭe, anyasya cha abhāvāṭ. (US II 109)

198 ṭaṭhāiveṭi. eṣā aviḍyā yannimiṭṭaḥ saṃsāro jāgraṭsvapnalakṣaṇaḥ. ṭasyā aviḍyāyāḥ viḍyā nivarṭikā. iṭyevam ṭvam abhayam prāpnoṣi. nāṭaḥ param jāgraṭsvapnaḍuḥkham anubhaviṣyasi, saṃsāraḍuḥkhān mukṭo'sīṭi. (US II 110)

199 Om iṭi. (US II 111)

200 anāṭmavasṭunaśchāsaṭṭvāṭ iṭi paramo heṭuḥ. (US III 116)

परमार्थदर्शननिष्ठेन त्यागः कर्तव्यः।[201] [US II 44]

APPENDIX C

Yoga Sutras of Patanjali

पातञ्जलयोगसूत्रम्

[pāṭañjalayogasūṭram]

QUARTER I

समाधि (Samadhi)

अथ योगानुशासनम्। [1] योगश्चित्तवृत्तिनिरोधः। [2] तदा द्रष्टुः स्वरूपेऽवस्थानम्। [3] वृत्तिसारूप्यमितरत्र। [4] वृत्तयः पञ्चतय्यः क्लिष्टाक्लिष्टाः। [5] प्रमाणविपर्ययविकल्पनिद्रास्मृतयः। [6] प्रत्यक्षानुमानागमाः प्रमाणानि। [7] विपर्ययो मिथ्याज्ञानमतद्रूपप्रतिष्ठम्। [8] शब्दज्ञानानुपाती वस्तुशून्यो विकल्पः। [9] अभावप्रत्ययालम्बना वृत्तिर्निद्रा। [10] अनुभूतविषयासम्प्रमोषः स्मृतिः। [11] अभ्यासवैराग्याभ्यां तन्निरोधः। [12] तत्र स्थितौ यत्नोऽभ्यासः। [13] स तु दीर्घकालनैरन्तर्यसत्कारासेवितो दृढभूमिः। [14] दृष्टानुश्रविकविषयवितृष्णस्य वशीकारसंज्ञा वैराग्यम्। [15] तत्परं पुरुषख्यातेर्गुणवैतृष्ण्यम्। [16] वितर्कविचारानन्दास्मितारूपानुगमात्सम्प्रज्ञातः। [17] विरामप्रत्ययाभ्यासपूर्वः संस्कारशेषोऽन्यः। [18] भवप्रत्ययो विदेहप्रकृतिलयानाम्। [19] श्रद्धावीर्यस्मृतिसमाधिप्रज्ञापूर्वक इतरेषाम्। [20] तीव्रसंवेगानामासन्नः। [21] मृदुमध्याधिमात्रत्वात्ततोऽपि विशेषः। [22] ईश्वरप्रणिधानाद्वा। [23] क्लेशकर्मविपाकाशयैरपरामृष्टः पुरुषविशेष ईश्वरः। [24] तत्र निरतिशयं सर्वज्ञबीजम्। [25] पूर्वेषामपि गुरुः कालेनानवच्छेदात्। [26] तस्य वाचकः प्रणवः। [27] तज्जपस्तदर्थभावनम्। [28] ततः प्रत्यक्चेतनाधिगमोऽप्यन्तरायाभावश्च। [29] व्याधिस्त्यानसंशयप्रमादालस्याविरतिभ्रान्तिदर्शनालब्धभूमिकत्वानवस्थितत्वानि चित्तविक्षेपास्तेऽन्तरायाः। [30] दुःखदौर्मनस्याङ्गमेजयत्वश्वासप्रश्वासा विक्षेपसहभुवः। [31]

---

201 ṭasmāḍ aviḍyākāryaṭvāṭ sarvakarmaṇām ṭaṭsāḍhanānām cha yajño-pavīṭāḍīnām paramārṭhaḍarśananiṣṭhena ṭyāgaḥ karṭavyaḥ. (US II 44)

तत्प्रतिषेधार्थमेकतत्त्वाभ्यासः। [32] मैत्रीकरुणामुदितोपेक्षाणां सुखदुःखपुण्यापुण्यविषयाणां भावनातश्चित्तप्रसादनम्। [33] प्रच्छर्दनविधारणाभ्यां वा प्राणस्य। [34] विषयवती वा प्रवृत्तिरुत्पन्ना मनसः स्थितिनिबन्धिनी। [35] विशोका वा ज्योतिष्मती। [36] वीतरागविषयं वा चित्तम्। [37] स्वप्ननिद्राज्ञानालम्बनं वा। [38] यथाभिमतध्यानाद्वा। [39] परमाणुपरममहत्त्वान्तोऽस्य वशीकारः। [40] क्षीणवृत्तेरभिजातस्येव मणेर्ग्रहीतृग्रहणग्राह्येषु तत्स्थतदञ्जनता समापत्तिः। [41] तत्र शब्दार्थज्ञानविकल्पैः सङ्कीर्णा सवितर्का समापत्तिः। [42] स्मृतिपरिशुद्धौ स्वरूपशून्येवार्थमात्रनिर्भासा निर्वितर्का। [43] एतयैव सविचारा निर्विचारा च सूक्ष्मविषया व्याख्याता। [44] सूक्ष्मविषयत्वं चालिङ्गपर्यवसानम्। [45] ता एव सबीजः समाधिः। [46] निर्विचारवैशारद्येऽध्यात्मप्रसादः। [47] ऋतम्भरा तत्र प्रज्ञा। [48] श्रुतानुमानप्रज्ञाभ्यामन्यविषया विशेषार्थत्वात्। [49] तज्जः संस्कारोऽन्यसंस्कारप्रतिबन्धी। [50] तस्यापि निरोधे सर्वनिरोधान्निर्बीजः समाधिः। [51]

aṭha yogānuśāsanam [1] yogaśchiṭṭavṛṭṭinirodhaḥ [2] ṭaḍā ḍraṣṭuḥ svarūpe'vasṭhānam [3] vṛṭṭisārūpyam iṭaraṭra [4] vṛṭṭayaḥ pañchaṭayyaḥ kliṣṭākliṣṭāḥ [5] pramāṇa viparyayavikalpaniḍrāsmṛṭayaḥ [6] praṭyakṣānumānāgamāḥ pramāṇāni [7] viparyayo miṭhyājñānam aṭaḍrūpapraṭiṣṭham [8] śabḍajñānānupāṭī vasṭuśunyo vikalpaḥ [9] abhāvapraṭyayālambanā vṛṭṭir niḍrā [10] anubhūṭaviṣayāsampramoṣaḥ smṛṭiḥ [11] abhyāsavāirāgyābhyām ṭannirodhaḥ [12] ṭaṭra sṭhiṭāu yaṭno'bhyāsaḥ [13] sa ṭu ḍīrghakālanāiranṭaryasaṭkārāseviṭo ḍṛdhabhūmiḥ [14] ḍṛṣṭānuśravikaviṣayaviṭṛṣṇasya vaśīkārasamjñā vāirāgyam [15] ṭaṭparam puruṣakhyāṭer guṇavāiṭṛṣṇyam [16] viṭarkavichārānanḍāsmiṭārūpānugamāṭ samprajñāṭaḥ [17] virāmapraṭyayābhyāsapūrvaḥ saṃskāraśeṣo'nyaḥ [18] bhavapraṭyayo viḍehaprakṛṭilayānām [19] śraḍḍhāvīryasmṛṭisamāḍhiprajñāpurvaka iṭareṣām [20] ṭīvrasaṃvegānāmāsannaḥ [21] mṛḍumaḍhyāḍhimāṭraṭvāṭṭaṭo'pi viśeṣaḥ [22] īśvarapraṇiḍhānāḍvā [23] kleśakarmavipākāśayāir aparāmṛṣṭaḥ puruṣaviśeṣa īśvaraḥ [24] ṭaṭra niraṭiśayam sarvajñabījam [25] pūrveṣāmapi guruḥ kālenānavachchheḍāṭ [26] ṭasya vāchakaḥ praṇavaḥ [27] ṭajjapas ṭaḍarṭhabhāvanam [28] ṭaṭaḥ praṭyakcheṭanāḍhigamo' pyanṭarāyābhāvaścha [29] vyāḍhisṭyānasaṃśayapramāḍālasyāviraṭibhrānṭiḍarśanālabḍhabhūmikaṭvā-navasṭhiṭaṭvāni chiṭṭavikṣepās ṭe'nṭarāyāḥ [30] ḍuḥkha-ḍāurmanasyāṅgamejayaṭvaśvāsapraśvāsā vikṣepasaha-bhuvaḥ [31] ṭaṭpraṭiṣeḍhārṭham ekaṭaṭṭvābhyāsaḥ [32] māiṭrīkaruṇāmuḍiṭopekṣāṇām sukhaḍuḥkhapuṇyāpuṇya-viṣayāṇām bhāvanāṭaś chiṭṭaprasāḍanam [33] prachchharḍanaviḍhāraṇābhyām vā prāṇasya [34] viṣayavaṭī vā pravṛṭṭir uṭpannā manasaḥ sṭhiṭinibanḍhinī [35] viśokā vā jyoṭiṣmaṭī [36] vīṭarāgaviṣayam vā chiṭṭam [37] svapnaniḍrājñānālambanam vā [38] yaṭhābhimaṭa-ḍhyānāḍ vā [39] paramāṇuparamamahaṭṭvānṭo'sya vaśīkāraḥ [40] kṣīṇavṛṭṭer abhijāṭasyeva maṇergrahīṭṛ-grahaṇagrāhyeṣu ṭaṭsṭhaṭaḍañjanaṭā samāpaṭṭiḥ [41] ṭaṭra śabḍārṭhajñānavikalpāiḥ saṅkīrṇā saviṭarkā samāpaṭṭiḥ [42] smṛṭipariśuḍḍhāu svarūpaśūnyevārṭhamāṭranirbhāsā nirviṭarkā [43] eṭyāiva savichārā nirvichārā cha sūkṣma-viṣayā vyākhyāṭā [44] sūkṣmaviṣayaṭvam chāliṅga-paryavasānam [45] ṭā eva sabījaḥ samāḍhiḥ [46] nirvichāra-vāiśāraḍye'ḍhyāṭmaprasāḍaḥ [47] ṛṭambharā ṭaṭra prajñā [48] śruṭānumānaprajñābhyām anyaviṣayā viśeṣārṭhaṭvāṭ [49] ṭajjaḥ saṃskāro'nyasaṃskārapraṭibanḍhī [50] ṭasyāpi niroḍhe sarvaniroḍhānnirbījaḥ samāḍhiḥ [51]

QUARTER II

साधन (Sadhana, Means)

तपःस्वाध्यायेश्वरप्रणिधानानि क्रियायोगः। [1] समाधिभावनार्थः क्लेशतनूकरणार्थश्च। [2] अविद्यास्मितारागद्वेषाभिनिवेशाः क्लेशाः। [3] अविद्याक्षेत्रमुत्तरेषां प्रसुप्ततनुविच्छिन्नोदाराणाम्। [4] अनित्याशुचिदुःखानात्मसु नित्यशुचिसुखात्मख्यातिरविद्या। [5] दृग्दर्शनशक्त्योरेकात्मतेवास्मिता। [6] सुखानुशयी रागः। [7] दुःखानुशयी द्वेषः। [8] स्वरसवाही विदुषोऽपि तथारूढोऽभिनिवेशः। [9] ते प्रतिप्रसवहेयाः सूक्ष्माः। [10] ध्यानहेयास्तद्वृत्तयः। [11] क्लेशमूलः कर्माशयो दृष्टादृष्टजन्मवेदनीयः। [12] सति मूले तद्विपाको जात्यायुर्भोगाः। [13] ते ह्लादपरितापफलाः पुण्यापुण्यहेतुत्वात्। [14] परिणामतापसंस्कारदुःखैर्गुणवृत्तिविरोधाच्च दुःखमेव सर्वं विवेकिनः। [15] हेयं दुःखमनागतम्। [16] द्रष्टृदृश्ययोः संयोगो हेयहेतुः। [17] प्रकाशक्रियास्थितिशीलं भूतेन्द्रियात्मकं भोगापवर्गार्थं दृश्यम्। [18] विशेषाविशेष-

लिङ्गमात्रालिङ्गानि गुणपर्वाणि। [19] द्रष्टा दृशिमात्रः शुद्धोऽपि प्रत्ययानुपश्यः। [20] तदर्थ एव दृश्यस्यात्मा। [21] कृतार्थं प्रति नष्टमप्यनष्टं तदन्यसाधारणत्वात्। [22] स्वस्वामिशक्त्योः स्वरूपोपलब्धिहेतुः संयोगः। [23] तस्य हेतुरविद्या। [24] तदभावात् संयोगाभावो हानं तद्दृशेः कैवल्यम्। [25] विवेकख्यातिरविप्लवा हानोपायः। [26] तस्य सप्तधा प्रान्तभूमिः प्रज्ञा। [27] योगाङ्गानुष्ठानादशुद्धिक्षये ज्ञानदीप्तिराविवेकख्यातेः। [28] यमनियमासनप्राणायामप्रत्याहारधारणाध्यानसमाधयोऽष्टावङ्गानि। [29] अहिंसासत्यास्तेयब्रह्मचर्यापरिग्रहा यमाः। [30] जातिदेशकालसमयानवच्छिन्नाः सार्वभौमा महाव्रतम्। [31] शौचसन्तोषतपःस्वाध्यायेश्वरप्रणिधानानि नियमाः। [32] वितर्कबाधने प्रतिपक्षभावनम्। [33] वितर्का हिंसादयः कृतकारितानुमोदिता लोभक्रोधमोहपूर्वका मृदुमध्याधिमात्रा दुःखाज्ञानानन्तफला इति प्रतिपक्षभावनम्। [34] अहिंसाप्रतिष्ठायां तत्सन्निधौ वैरत्यागः। [35] सत्यप्रतिष्ठायां क्रियाफलाश्रयत्वम्। [36] अस्तेयप्रतिष्ठायां सर्वरत्नोपस्थानम्। [37] ब्रह्मचर्यप्रतिष्ठायां वीर्यलाभः। [38] अपरिग्रहस्थैर्ये जन्मकथंतासंबोधः। [39] शौचात्स्वाङ्गजुगुप्सा परैरसंसर्गः। [40] सत्त्वशुद्धिसौमनस्यैकाग्र्येन्द्रियजयात्मदर्शनयोग्यत्वानि च। [41] सन्तोषादनुत्तमसुखलाभः। [42] कायेन्द्रियसिद्धिरशुद्धिक्षयात्तपसः। [43] स्वाध्यायादिष्टदेवतासम्प्रयोगः। [44] समाधिसिद्धिरीश्वरप्रणिधानात्। [45] स्थिरसुखमासनम्। [46] प्रयत्नशैथिल्यानन्त्यसमापत्तिभ्याम्। [47] ततो द्वन्द्वानभिघातः। [48] तस्मिन्सति श्वासप्रश्वासयोर्गतिविच्छेदः प्राणायामः। [49] बाह्याभ्यन्तरस्तम्भवृत्तिर्देशकालसङ्ख्याभिः परिदृष्टो दीर्घसूक्ष्मः। [50] बाह्याभ्यन्तरविषयाक्षेपी चतुर्थः। [51] ततः क्षीयते प्रकाशावरणम्। [52] धारणासु च योग्यता मनसः। [53] स्वविषयासम्प्रयोगे चित्तस्य स्वरूपानुकार इवेन्द्रियाणां प्रत्याहारः। [54] ततः परमा वश्यतेन्द्रियाणाम्। [55]

ṭapaḥsvāḍhyāyeśvarapraṇiḍhānāni kriyāyogaḥ [1] samāḍhibhāvanārṭhaḥ kleśaṭanūkaraṇārṭhaś cha [2] aviḍyāsmiṭārāgaḍveṣābhiniveśāḥ kleśāḥ [3] aviḍyākṣeṭram uṭṭareṣām prasupṭaṭanuvichchhinnoḍārāṇām [4] aniṭyāśuchiḍuḥkhānāṭmasu niṭyaśuchisukhāṭmakhyāṭir aviḍyā [5] ḍṛgḍarśanaśakṭyorekāṭmaṭevāsmiṭā [6] sukhānuśayī rāgaḥ [7] ḍuḥkhānuśayī ḍveṣaḥ [8] svarasavāhī viḍuṣo'pi ṭaṭhārūḍho'bhiniveśaḥ [9] ṭe praṭiprasavaheyāḥ sūkṣmāḥ [10] ḍhyānaheyāsṭaḍvṛṭṭayaḥ [11] kleśamūlaḥ karmāśayo ḍṛṣṭāḍṛṣṭajanmaveḍanīyaḥ [12] saṭi mūle ṭaḍvipāko jāṭyāyurbhogāḥ [13] ṭe hlāḍapariṭāpaphalāḥ puṇyāpuṇyaheṭuṭvāṭ [14] pariṇāmaṭāpasaṃskāraḍuḥkhāirguṇavṛṭṭiviroḍhāchcha ḍuḥkhameva sarvam vivekinaḥ [15] heyam ḍuḥkham anāgaṭam [16] ḍraṣṭṛḍṛśyayoḥ saṃyogo heyaheṭuḥ [17] prakāśakriyāsṭhiṭiśīlam bhūṭenḍriyāṭmakam bhogāpavargārṭham ḍṛśyam [18] viśeṣāviśeṣaliṅgamāṭrāliṅgāni guṇaparvāṇi [19] ḍraṣṭā ḍṛśimāṭraḥ śuḍḍho'pi praṭyayānupaśyaḥ [20] ṭaḍarṭha eva ḍṛśyasyāṭmā [21] kṛṭārṭham praṭi naṣṭamapyanaṣṭam ṭaḍanyasāḍhāraṇaṭvāṭ [22] svasvāmiśakṭyoḥ svarūpopalabḍhiheṭuḥ saṃyogaḥ [23] ṭasya heṭuraviḍyā [24] ṭaḍabhāvāṭ saṃyogābhāvo hānam ṭaḍḍṛśeḥ kāivalyam [25] vivekakhyāṭir aviplavā hānopāyaḥ [26] ṭasya sapṭaḍhā prānṭabhūmiḥ prajñā [27] yogāṅgānuṣṭhānāḍaśuḍḍhikṣaye jñānaḍīpṭir āvivekakhyāṭeḥ [28] yamaniyamāsanaprāṇāyāmapraṭyāhāraḍhāraṇāḍhyānasamāḍhayo'ṣṭāvaṅgāni [29] ahiṃsāsaṭyāsṭeyabrahmacharyāparigrahā yamāḥ [30] jāṭiḍeśakālasamayānavachchhinnāḥ sārvabhāumā mahāvraṭam [31] śāuchasanṭoṣaṭapaḥsvāḍhyāyeśvarapraṇiḍhānāni niyamāḥ [32] viṭarkabāḍhane praṭipakṣabhāvanam [33] viṭarkā hiṃsāḍayaḥ kṛṭakāriṭānumoḍiṭā lobhakroḍhamohapūrvakā mṛḍumaḍhyāḍhimāṭrā ḍuḥkhājñānānanṭaphalā iṭi praṭipakṣabhāvanam [34] ahiṃsāpraṭiṣṭhāyām ṭaṭsanniḍhāu vāiraṭyāgaḥ [35] saṭyapraṭiṣṭhāyām kriyāphalāśrayaṭvam [36] asṭeyapraṭiṣṭhāyām sarvaraṭnopasṭhānam [37] brahmacharyapraṭiṣṭhāyām vīryalābhaḥ [38] aparigrahasṭhāirye janmakaṭhanṭāsamboḍhaḥ [39] śāuchāṭ svāṅgajugupsā parāir asaṃsargaḥ [40] saṭṭvaśuḍḍhisāumanasyāikāgryenḍriyajayāṭmaḍarśanayogyaṭvāni cha [41] sanṭoṣāḍ anuṭṭamasukhalābhaḥ [42] kāyenḍriyasiḍḍhir aśuḍḍhikṣayāṭṭapasaḥ [43] svāḍhyāyāḍ iṣṭaḍevaṭāsamprayogaḥ [44] samāḍhisiḍḍhir īśvarapraṇiḍhānāṭ [45] sṭhirasukham āsanam [46] prayaṭnaśāiṭhilyānanṭyasamāpaṭṭibhyām [47] ṭaṭo ḍvanḍvānabhighāṭaḥ [48] ṭasmin saṭi śvāsapraśvāsayor gaṭivichchheḍaḥ prāṇāyāmaḥ [49] bāhyābhyanṭarasṭambhavṛṭṭir ḍeśakālasaṅkhyābhiḥ pariḍṛṣto ḍīrghasūkṣmaḥ [50] bāhyābhyanṭaraviṣayākṣepī chaṭurṭhaḥ [51] ṭaṭaḥ kṣīyaṭe prakāśāvaraṇam [52] ḍhāraṇāsu cha yogyaṭā manasaḥ [53] svaviṣayāsamprayoge chiṭṭasya svarūpānūkāra ivendriyāṇām pratyāhāraḥ [54] ṭaṭaḥ paramā vaśyaṭendriyāṇām [55]

QUARTER III

विभूति (Vibhuti, Glory)

देशबन्धश्चित्तस्य धारणा। [1] तत्र प्रत्ययैकतानता ध्यानम्। [2] तदेवार्थमात्रनिर्भासं स्वरूपशून्यमिव समाधिः। [3] त्रयमेकत्र संयमः। [4] तज्जयात्प्रज्ञालोकः। [5] तस्य भूमिषु विनियोगः। [6] त्रयमन्तरङ्गं पूर्वेभ्यः। [7] तदपि बहिरङ्गं निर्बीजस्य। [8] व्युत्थाननिरोधसंस्कारयोरभिभवप्रादुर्भावौ निरोधक्षणचित्तान्वयो निरोधपरिणामः। [9] तस्य प्रशान्तवाहिता संस्कारात्। [10] सर्वार्थतैकाग्रतयोः क्षयोदयौ चित्तस्य समाधिपरिणामः। [11] ततः पुनः शान्तोदितौ तुल्यप्रत्ययौ चित्तस्यैकाग्रतापरिणामः। [12] एतेन भूतेन्द्रियेषु धर्मलक्षणावस्थापरिणामा व्याख्याताः। [13] शान्तोदिताव्यपदेश्यधर्मानुपाती धर्मी। [14] क्रमान्यत्वं परिणामान्यत्वे हेतुः। [15] परिणामत्रय-संयमादतीतानागतज्ञानम्। [16] शब्दार्थप्रत्ययानामितरेतराध्यासात् सङ्करस्तत्प्रविभागसंयमात् सर्वभूतरुतज्ञानम्। [17] संस्कार-साक्षात्करणात्पूर्वजातिज्ञानम्। [18] प्रत्ययस्य परचित्तज्ञानम्। [19] न च तत्सालम्बनं तस्याविषयीभूतत्वात्। [20] कायरूपसंयमात्तद्ग्राह्यशक्तिस्तम्भे चक्षुःप्रकाशासम्प्रयोगेऽन्तर्धानम्। [21] सोपक्रमं निरुपक्रमं च कर्म तत्संयमादपरान्तज्ञानमरिष्टेभ्यो वा। [22] मैत्र्यादिषु बलानि। [23] बलेषु हस्तिबलादीनि। [24] प्रवृत्त्या लोकन्यासात्सूक्ष्मव्यवहितविप्रकृष्टज्ञानम्। [25] भुवनज्ञानं सूर्ये संयमात्। [26] चन्द्रे ताराव्यूहज्ञानम्। [27] ध्रुवे तद्गतिज्ञानम्। [28] नाभिचक्रे कायव्यूहज्ञानम्। [29] कण्ठकूपे क्षुत्पिपासानिवृत्तिः। [30] कूर्मनाड्यां स्थैर्यम्। [31] मूर्धज्योतिषि सिद्धदर्शनम्। [32] प्रातिभाद्वा सर्वम्। [33] हृदये चित्तसंवित्। [34] सत्त्वपुरुषयोरत्यन्तासङ्कीर्णयोः प्रत्ययाविशेषो भोगः परार्थत्वात्स्वार्थसंयमात् पुरुषज्ञानम्। [35] ततः प्रातिभश्रावण-वेदनादर्शास्वादवार्ता जायन्ते। [36] ते समाधावुपसर्गा व्युत्थाने सिद्धयः। [37] बन्धकारणशैथिल्यात्प्रचारसंवेदनाच्च चित्तस्य परशरीरावेशः। [38] उदानजयाज्जलपङ्ककण्टकादिष्वसङ्ग उत्क्रान्तिश्च। [39] समानजया-ज्ज्वलनम्। [40] श्रोत्राकाशयोः सम्बन्धसंयमाद्दिव्यं श्रोत्रम्। [41]

कायाकाशयोः सम्बन्धसंयमाल्लघुतूलसमापत्तेश्चाकाशगमनम्। [42] बहिरकल्पिता वृत्तिर्महाविदेहा ततः प्रकाशावरणक्षयः। [43] स्थूलस्वरूपसूक्ष्मान्वयार्थवत्त्वसंयमाद्भूतजयः। [44] ततोऽणिमादिप्रादुर्भावः कायसम्पत्तद्धर्मानभिघातश्च। [45] रूपलावण्यबलवज्रसंहननत्वानि कायसम्पत्। [46] ग्रहणस्वरूपास्मितान्वयार्थवत्त्वसंयमादिन्द्रियजयः। [47] ततो मनोजवित्वं विकरणभावः प्रधानजयश्च। [48] सत्त्वपुरुषान्यताख्यातिमात्रस्य सर्वभावाधिष्ठातृत्वं सर्वज्ञातृत्वं च। [49] तद्वैराग्यादपि दोषबीजक्षये कैवल्यम्। [50] स्थान्युपनिमन्त्रणे सङ्गस्मयाकरणं पुनरनिष्टप्रसङ्गात्। [51] क्षणतत्क्रमयोः संयमाद्विवेकजं ज्ञानम्। [52] जातिलक्षणदेशैरन्यतानवच्छेदात् तुल्ययोस्ततः प्रतिपत्तिः। [53] तारकं सर्वविषयं सर्वथाविषयमक्रमं चेति विवेकजं ज्ञानम्। [54] सत्त्वपुरुषयोः शुद्धिसाम्ये कैवल्यम्। [55]

ḍeśabanḍhaś chiṭṭasya ḍhāraṇā [1] ṭaṭra praṭyayāikaṭānaṭā ḍhyānam [2] ṭaḍevārṭhamāṭranirbhāsam svarūpaśūnyamiva samāḍhiḥ [3] ṭrayam ekaṭra saṃyamaḥ [4] ṭajjayāṭ prajñālokaḥ [5] ṭasya bhūmiṣu viniyogaḥ [6] ṭrayam anṭaraṅgam pūrvebhyaḥ [7] ṭaḍapi bahiraṅgam nirbījasya [8] vyuṭṭhānaniroḍhasaṃskārayor abhibhavaprāḍurbhāvāu niroḍhakṣaṇachiṭṭānvayo niroḍhapariṇāmaḥ [9] ṭasya praśānṭavāhiṭā saṃskārāṭ [10] sarvārṭhaṭāikāgraṭayoḥ kṣayoḍayāu chiṭṭasya samāḍhipariṇāmaḥ [11] ṭaṭaḥ punaḥ śānṭoḍiṭāu ṭulyapraṭyayāu chiṭṭasyāikāgraṭāpariṇāmaḥ [12] eṭena bhūṭenḍriyeṣu ḍharmalakṣaṇāvasṭhāpariṇāmā vyākhyāṭāḥ [13] śānṭoḍiṭāvyapaḍeśyaḍharmānupāṭī ḍharmī [14] kramānyaṭvam pariṇāmānyaṭve heṭuḥ [15] pariṇāmaṭrayasaṃyamāḍ aṭīṭānāgaṭajñānam [16] śabḍārṭhapraṭyayānāmiṭareṭarāḍhyāsāṭ saṅkaras ṭaṭpravibhāgasaṃyamāṭ sarvabhūṭaruṭajñānam [17] saṃskārasākṣāṭkaraṇāṭ pūrvajāṭijñānam [18] praṭyayasya parachiṭṭajñānam [19] na cha ṭaṭsālambanam ṭasyāviṣayībhūṭaṭvāṭ [20] kāyarūpasaṃyamāṭ ṭaḍgrāhyaśakṭisṭambhe chakṣuḥprakāśāsamprayoge'nṭarḍhānam [21] sopakramam nirupakramam cha karma ṭaṭsaṃyamāḍaparānṭajñānamariṣṭebhyo vā [22] māiṭryāḍiṣu balāni [23] baleṣu hasṭibalāḍīni [24] pravṛṭṭyā lokanyāsāṭ sūkṣmavyavahiṭaviprakṛṣṭajñānam [25] bhuvanajñānam sūrye saṃyamāṭ [26] chanḍre ṭārāvyūhajñānam [27] ḍhruve ṭaḍgaṭijñānam [28] nābhichakre kāyavyūhajñānam [29] kaṇṭhakūpe kṣuṭpipāsānivṛṭṭiḥ [30] kūrmanāḍyām sṭhāiryam [31] mūrḍhajyoṭiṣi siḍḍhaḍarśanam [32] prāṭibhāḍ vā sarvam [33] hṛḍaye chiṭṭasaṃviṭ [34] saṭṭvapuruṣayoraṭyanṭāsaṅkīrṇayoḥ praṭyayāviśeṣo bhogaḥ parārṭhaṭvāṭ svārṭhasaṃyamāṭ puruṣajñānam [35] ṭaṭaḥ prāṭibhaśrāvaṇaveḍanāḍarśāsvāḍavārṭā jāyanṭe [36] ṭe samāḍhāvupasargā vyuṭṭhāne siḍḍhayaḥ [37] banḍhakāraṇaśāiṭhilyāṭ prachārasaṃveḍanāchcha chiṭṭasya paraśarīrāveśaḥ [38] uḍānajayājjalapaṅkakaṇṭakāḍiṣvasaṅga uṭkrānṭiścha [39] samānajayājjvalanam [40] śroṭrākāśayoḥ sambanḍhasaṃyamāḍḍivyam śroṭram [41] kāyākāśayoḥ sambanḍhasaṃyamāllaghuṭūlasamāpaṭṭeśchākāśagamanam [42] bahirakalpiṭā vṛṭṭir mahāviḍehā ṭaṭaḥ prakāśāvaraṇakṣayaḥ [43] sṭhūlasvarūpasūkṣmānvayārṭhavaṭṭvasaṃyamāḍ bhūṭajayaḥ [44] ṭaṭo'ṇimāḍiprāḍurbhāvaḥ kāyasampaṭ ṭaḍḍharmānabhighāṭaścha [45] rūpalāvaṇyabalavajrasaṃhananaṭvāni kāyasampaṭ [46] grahaṇasvarūpāsmiṭānvayārṭhavaṭṭvasaṃyamāḍ inḍriyajayaḥ [47] ṭaṭo manojaviṭvam vikaraṇabhāvaḥ praḍhānajayaścha [48] saṭṭvapuruṣānyaṭākhyāṭimāṭrasya sarvabhāvāḍhiṣthāṭṛṭvam sarvajñāṭṛṭvañcha [49] ṭaḍvāirāgyāḍapi ḍoṣabījakṣaye kāivalyam [50] sṭhānyupanimanṭraṇe saṅgasmayākaraṇam punaraniṣṭaprasaṅgāṭ [51] kṣaṇaṭaṭkramayoḥ saṃyamāḍvivekajam jñānam [52] jāṭilakṣaṇaḍeśāiranyaṭānavachchheḍāṭ ṭulyayos ṭaṭaḥ praṭipaṭṭiḥ [53] ṭārakam sarvaviṣayam sarvaṭhāviṣayamakramam cheṭi vivekajam jñānam [54] saṭṭvapuruṣayoḥ śuḍḍhisāmye kāivalyam [55]

QUARTER IV

कैवल्य (Kaivalya)

जन्मौषधिमन्त्रतपःसमाधिजाः सिद्धयः। [1] जात्यन्तरपरिणामः प्रकृत्यापूरात्। [2] निमित्तमप्रयोजकं प्रकृतीनां वरणभेदस्तु ततः क्षेत्रिकवत्। [3] निर्माणचित्तान्यस्मितामात्रात्। [4] प्रवृत्तिभेदे प्रयोजकं चित्तमेकमनेकेषाम्। [5] तत्र ध्यानजमनाशयम्। [6] कर्माशुक्लाकृष्णं योगिनस्त्रिविधमितरेषाम्। [7] ततस्तद्विपाकानुगुणानामेवाभिव्यक्तिर्वासनानाम्। [8] जातिदेशकालव्यवहितानामप्यानन्तर्यं स्मृतिसंस्कारयोरेकरूपत्वात्। [9] तासामनादित्वं चाशिषो नित्यत्वात्। [10] हेतुफलाश्रयालम्बनैः संगृहीतत्वादेषामभावे तदभावः। [11] अतीतानागतं स्वरूपतोऽस्त्यध्वभेदाद्धर्माणाम्। [12] ते व्यक्तसूक्ष्मा

गुणात्मानः। [13] परिणामैकत्वाद्वस्तुतत्त्वम्। [14] वस्तुसाम्ये चित्तभेदात्तयोर्विभक्तः पन्थाः। [15] न चैकचित्ततन्त्रं वस्तु तदप्रमाणकं तदा किं स्यात्। [16] तदुपरागापेक्षित्वाच्चित्तस्य वस्तु ज्ञाताज्ञातम्। [17] सदा ज्ञाताश्चित्तवृत्तयस्तत्प्रभोः पुरुषस्यापरिणामित्वात्। [18] न तत्स्वाभासं दृश्यत्वात्। [19] एकसमये चोभयानवधारणम्। [20] चित्तान्तरदृश्ये बुद्धिबुद्धेरतिप्रसङ्गः स्मृतिसङ्करश्च। [21] चितेरप्रतिसङ्क्रमायास्तदाकारापत्तौ स्वबुद्धिसंवेदनम्। [22] द्रष्टृदृश्योपरक्तं चित्तं सर्वार्थम्। [23] तदसङ्ख्येयवासनाभिश्चित्रमपि परार्थं संहत्यकारित्वात्। [24] विशेषदर्शिन आत्मभावभावनाविनिवृत्तिः। [25] तदा विवेकनिम्नं कैवल्यप्राग्भारं चित्तम्। [26] तच्छिद्रेषु प्रत्ययान्तराणि संस्कारेभ्यः। [27] हानमेषां क्लेशवदुक्तम्। [28] प्रसङ्ख्यानेऽप्यकुसीदस्य सर्वथा विवेकख्यातेर्धर्ममेघः समाधिः। [29] ततः क्लेशकर्मनिवृत्तिः। [30] तदा सर्वावरणमलापेतस्य ज्ञानस्यानन्त्या-ज्ज्ञेयमल्पम्। [31] ततः कृतार्थानां परिणामक्रमसमाप्तिर्गुणानाम्। [32] क्षणप्रतियोगी परिणामापरान्तनिर्ग्राह्यः क्रमः। [33] पुरुषार्थशून्यानां गुणानां प्रतिप्रसवः कैवल्यं स्वरूपप्रतिष्ठा चितिशक्तिरिति॥ [34]

janmāuṣaḍhimanṭraṭapaḥsamāḍhijāḥ siḍḍhayaḥ [1] jāṭyanṭarapariṇāmaḥ prakṛṭyāpūrāṭ [2] nimiṭṭam aprayojakam prakṛṭīnām varaṇabheḍasṭu ṭaṭaḥ kṣeṭrikavaṭ [3] nirmāṇachiṭṭānyasmiṭāmāṭrāṭ [4] pravṛṭṭibheḍe prayojakam chiṭṭam ekamanekeṣām [5] ṭaṭra ḍhyānajam anāśayam [6] karmāśuklākṛṣṇam yoginas ṭriviḍham iṭareṣām [7] ṭaṭas ṭaḍvipākānuguṇānām evābhivyakṭir vāsanānām [8] jāṭiḍeśakālavyavahiṭānām apyānanṭaryam smṛṭisaṃskārayor ekarūpaṭvāṭ [9] ṭāsām anāḍiṭvam chāśiṣo niṭyaṭvāṭ [10] heṭuphalāśrayālambanāiḥ saṃgṛhīṭaṭvāḍ eṣāmabhāve ṭaḍabhāvaḥ [11] aṭīṭānāgaṭam svarūpaṭo' sṭyaḍhvabheḍāḍ ḍharmāṇām [12] ṭe vyakṭasūkṣmā guṇāṭmānaḥ [13] pariṇāmāikaṭvāḍ vasṭuṭaṭṭvam [14] vasṭusāmye chiṭṭabheḍāṭ ṭayorvibhakṭaḥ panṭhāḥ [15] na chāikachiṭṭaṭanṭram vasṭu ṭaḍapramāṇakam ṭaḍā kim syāṭ [16] ṭaḍuparāgāpekṣiṭvāchchiṭṭasya vasṭu jñāṭājñāṭam [17] saḍā jñāṭāśchiṭṭavṛṭṭayas ṭaṭprabhoḥ puruṣasyāpari-ṇāmiṭvāṭ [18] na ṭaṭsvābhāsam ḍṛśyaṭvāṭ [19] ekasamaye chobhayānavaḍhāraṇam [20] chiṭṭānṭaraḍṛśye buḍḍhi-buḍḍher aṭiprasaṅgaḥ smṛṭisaṅkaraścha [21] chiṭerapraṭi-saṅkramāyās ṭaḍākārāpaṭṭāu svabuḍḍhisaṃveḍanam [22] ḍraṣṭṛḍṛśyoparakṭam chiṭṭam sarvārṭham [23] ṭaḍasaṅkhyeyavāsanābhiś chiṭramapi parārṭham saṃhaṭya-kāriṭvāṭ [24] viśeṣaḍarśina āṭmabhāvabhāvanāvinivṛṭṭiḥ [25] ṭaḍā vivekanimnam kāivalyaprāgbhāram chiṭṭam [26] ṭachchhiḍreṣu praṭyayānṭarāṇi saṃskārebhyaḥ [27] hānameṣām kleśavaḍukṭam [28] prasaṅkhyāne' pyakusīḍasya sarvaṭhā vivekakhyāṭer ḍharmameghaḥ samāḍhiḥ [29] ṭaṭaḥ kleśakarmanivṛṭṭiḥ [30] ṭaḍā sarvāvaraṇamalāpeṭasya jñānasyānanṭyājjñeyamalpam [31] ṭaṭaḥ kṛṭārṭhānām pariṇāmakramasamāpṭir guṇānām [32] kṣaṇapraṭiyogī pariṇāmāparānṭanirgrāhyaḥ kramaḥ [33] puruṣārṭhaśūnyānām guṇānām praṭiprasavaḥ kāivalyam svarūpapraṭiṣṭhā chiṭiśakṭir iṭi [34]

APPENDIX E

Bibliography

YOGA PHILOSOPHY

1. The Brihadaranyka Upanishad
2. The Mandukya Upanishad
3. The Isha Upanishad
4. The Bhagavad Gita
5. Hindu Scriptures, by R.C. Zaehner [It has English translation of all the above four and many others.]
6. Upadesasahasri, by philosopher Shankara [I consulted one published by Sri Ramakrishna Math.]
7. Yoga Pradeep, of Gita Press, Gorakhpur, India [It has an exhaustive information on yoga and sutras.]

YOGA EXERCISES

1. YOGA Mind & Body, of Sivananda Yoga Vedanta Centre
2. The Yoga Handbook, by Noa Belling

www.ingramcontent.com/pod-product-compliance
Lightning Source LLC
Chambersburg PA
CBHW061402280526
45784CB00001B/347